Limb Amputation

Edited by Masaki Fujioka

Published in London, United Kingdom

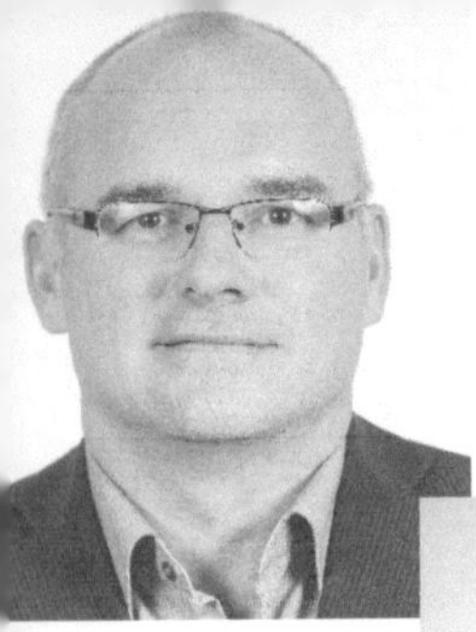
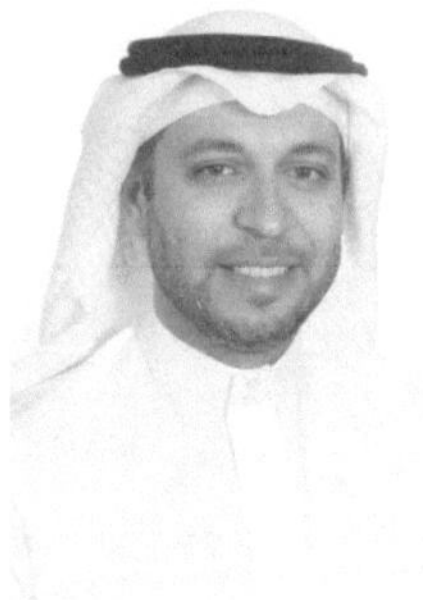
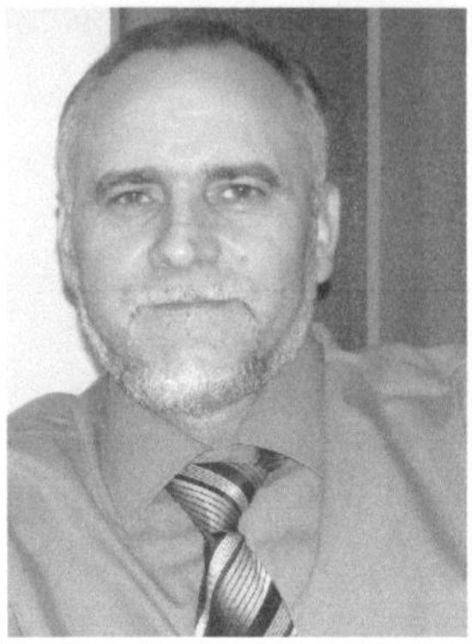
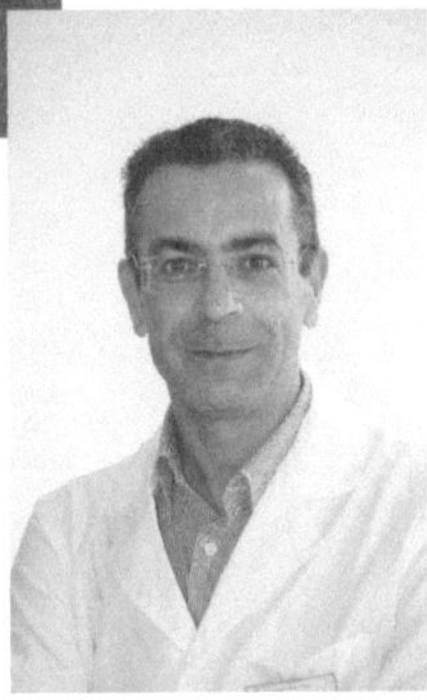
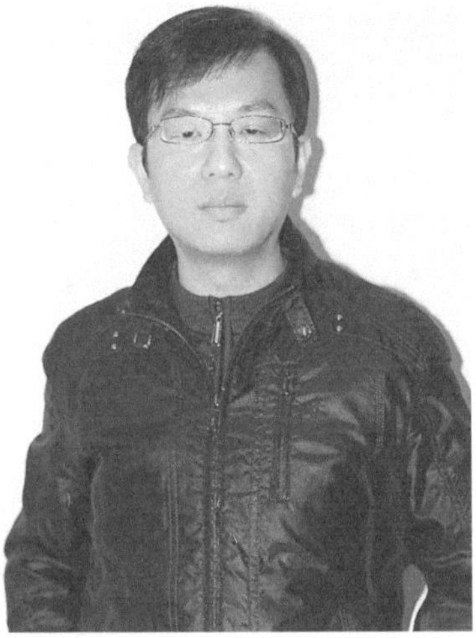
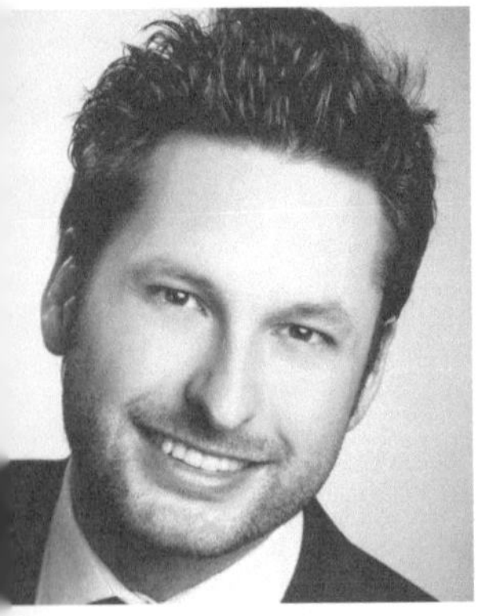
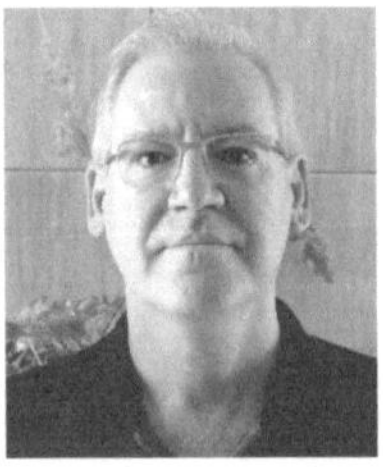

IntechOpen

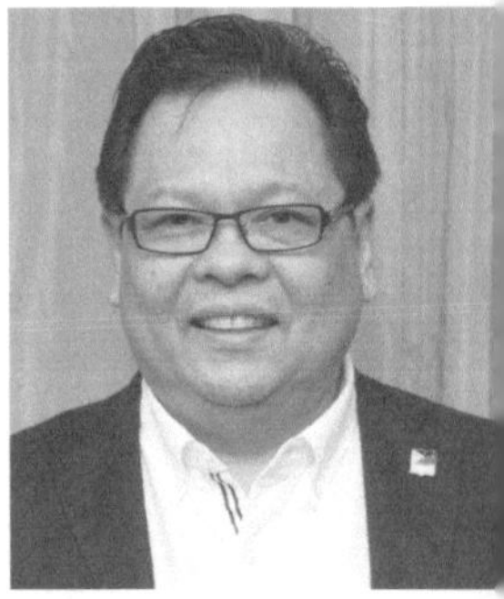
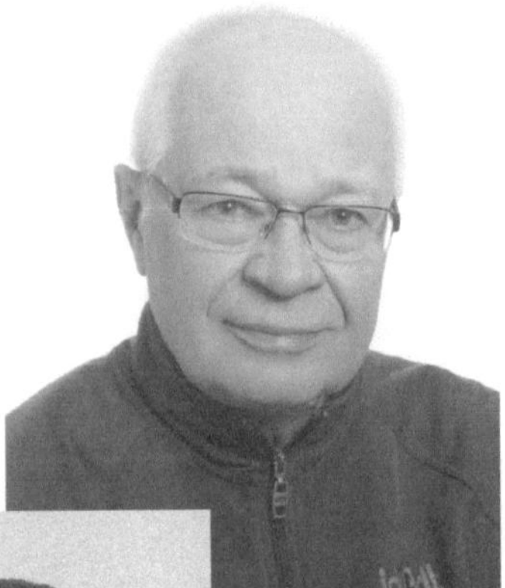
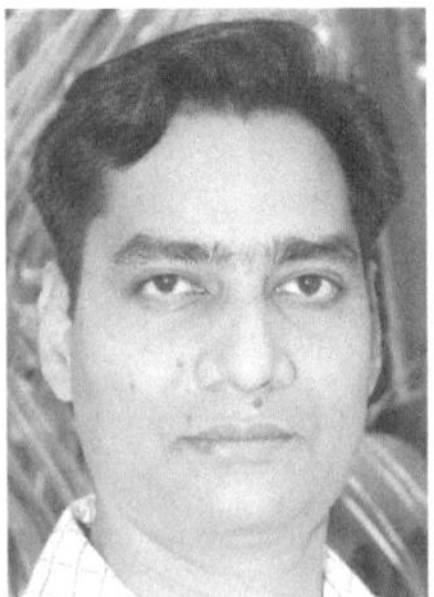
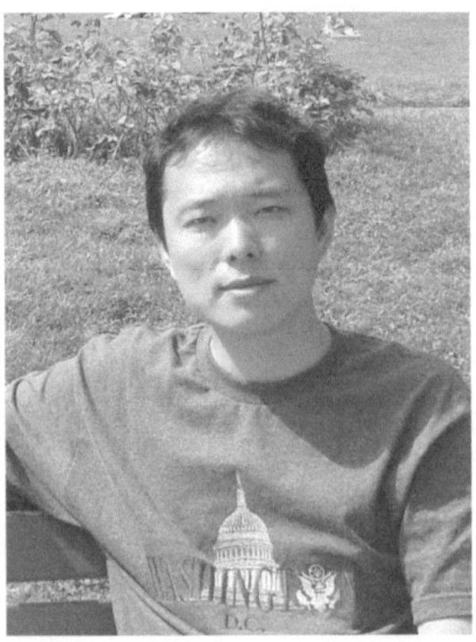
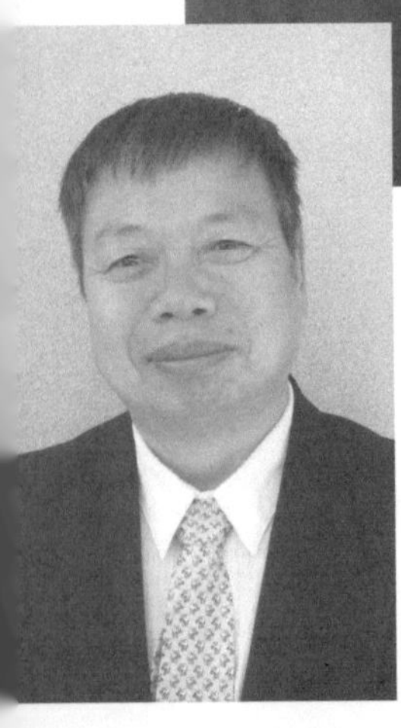
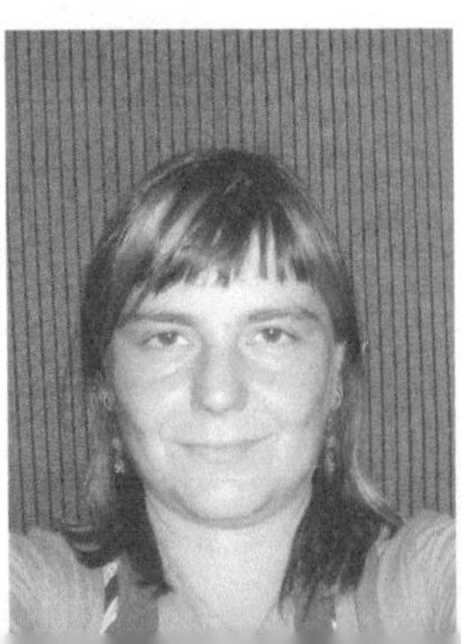

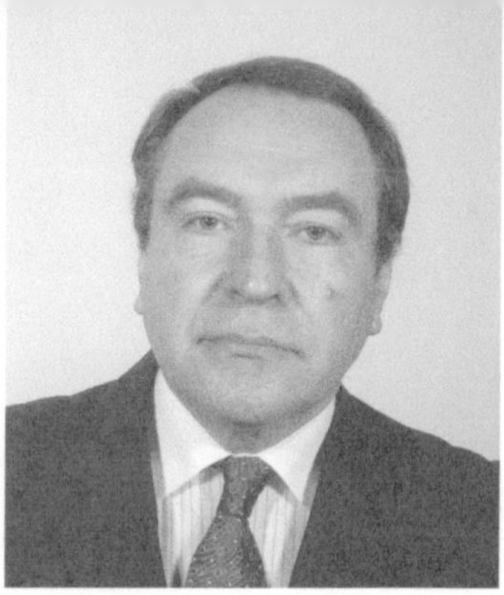
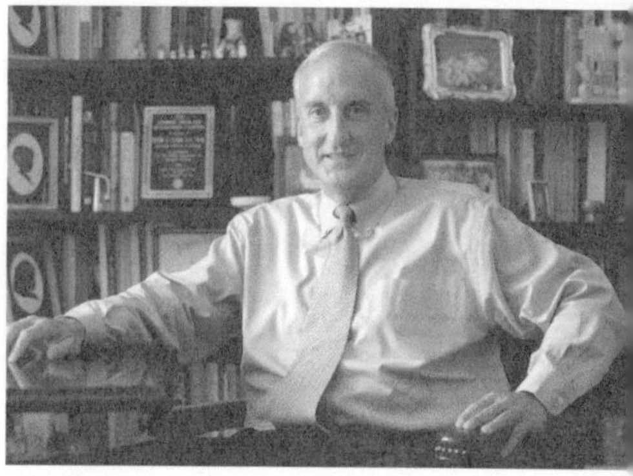
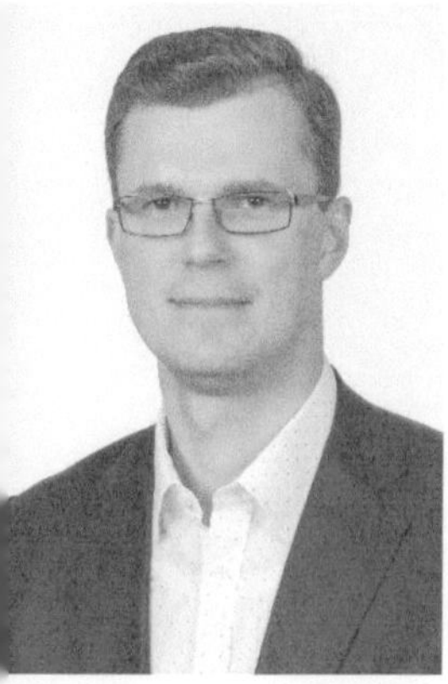
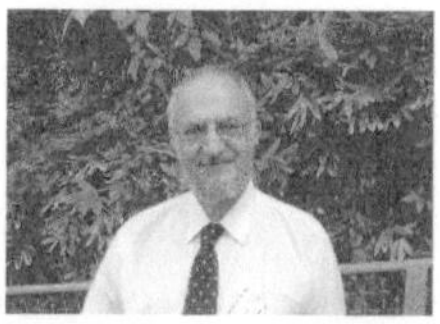
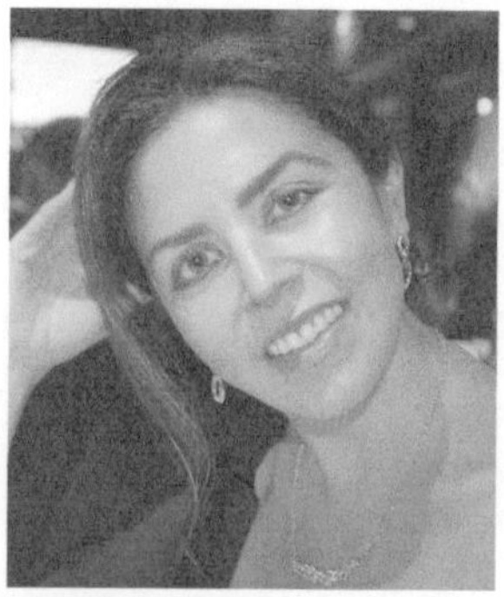

Supporting open minds since 2005

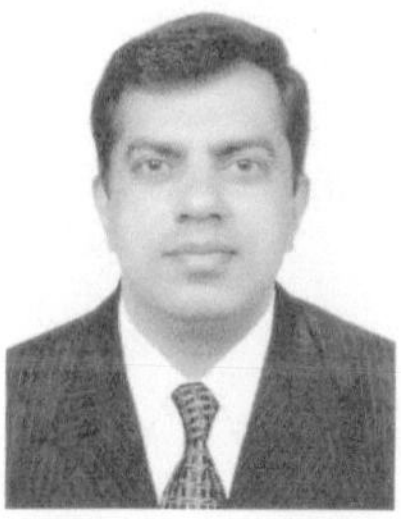
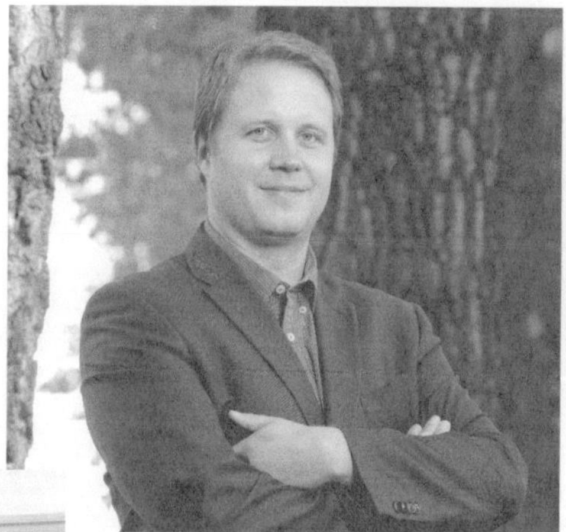
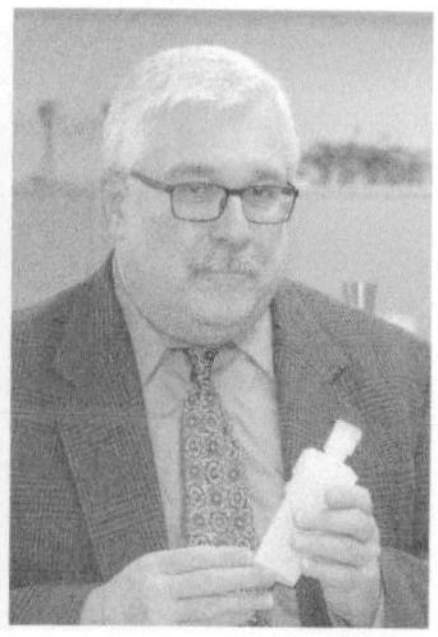
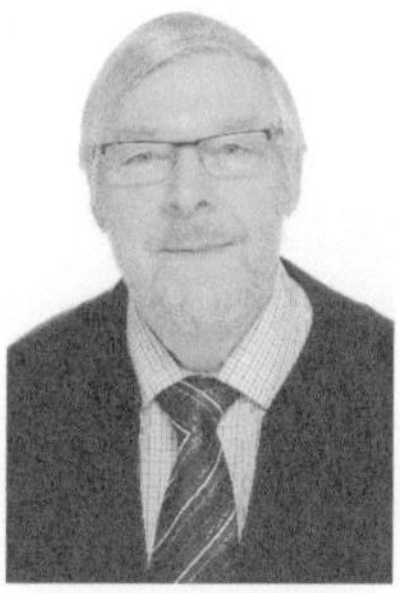
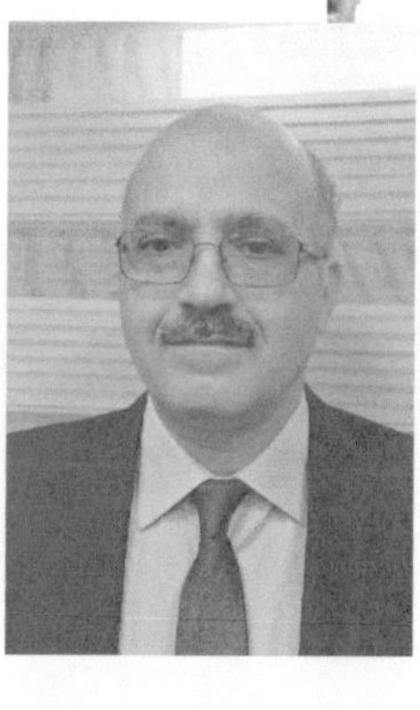
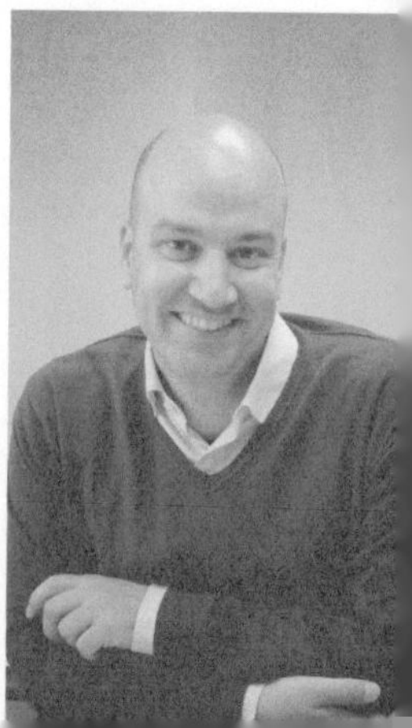
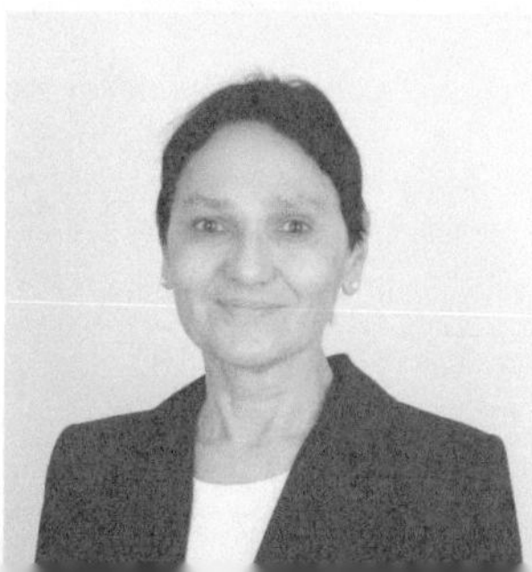

Limb Amputation
http://dx.doi.org/10.5772/intechopen.77805
Edited by Masaki Fujioka

Contributors
Masaki Fujioka, Isil Akgun Demir, Semra Karsidag, Mitsuru Nemoto, Rami Jahmani, Dror Paley

First published in London, United Kingdom, 2020 by IntechOpen
IntechOpen is the global imprint of INTECHOPEN LIMITED, registered in England and Wales, registration number: 11086078, 7th floor, 10 Lower Thames Street, London, EC3R 6AF, United Kingdom
Printed in Croatia

British Library Cataloguing-in-Publication Data
A catalogue record for this book is available from the British Library

Additional hard and PDF copies can be obtained from orders@intechopen.com

Limb Amputation
Edited by Masaki Fujioka
p. cm.
Print ISBN 978-1-78984-405-4
Online ISBN 978-1-78984-406-1
eBook (PDF) ISBN 978-1-83880-763-4

Meet the editor

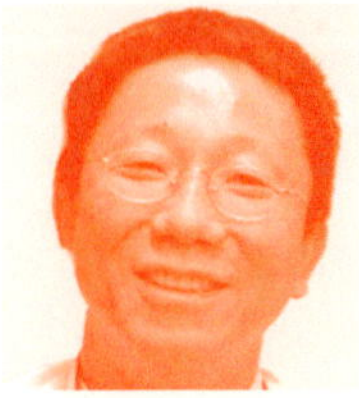

Masaki Fujioka is currently a Clinical Professor at the Department of Plastic and Reconstructive Surgery (PRS), at the Faculty of Medicine, Nagasaki University (2011-2020). He is also a Director of the Functional Form Research Section, Division of Functional Reconstructive Surgery (2019-2020), and Director of the Department of PRS (2003-2020), National Hospital Organization Nagasaki Medical Center. He was born in Shimonoseki city, Japan in 1961. He graduated in 1985 from the Jichi Medical School-Six Year Medical Program, and received his MD (PhD) degree from the Nagasaki University in 1998. Masaki Fujioka has authored more than 200 scientific papers and edited journals on the topics of microsurgical surgery, maxillofacial surgery, wound healing, and severe trauma.

Contents

Preface

Limb amputation is, in a sense, a physician's defeat in treating limb illness or injury. Patients often need to have limbs amputated to save them from advanced malignant neoplasms and severe limb infections, or due to the failure to repair severe limb trauma. However, efforts should be made to maintain limbs where possible and to minimize loss of function, even if amputation is required. We provide the latest developments in limb amputation for this purpose.

Cases of limb amputation may vary in the environment of each area, including war wounds from the battle field, infection and animal bites in developing countries, and traffic accidents and adult disease in advanced countries. At first, I present general remarks regarding limb amputations in the Introductory Chapter.

In the second chapter, I describe the treatment of peripheral arterial diseases and diabetes, which are the most common causes of amputation. Many patients with adult diseases such as peripheral arterial disease and diabetes require amputation, but patients always desire minimal amputation. Patients who undergo minor amputation can walk on their own feet; however, those with major amputation require an artificial leg, which impairs their activities. The aim of second chapter is to describe factors that lead to amputation, and propose a management plan to prevent major amputation.

Next is the topic of patients who need an amputation due to injuries to severe extremities. Multidisciplinary management of severe extremity injuries and appropriate wound assessment can not only save the patient's life but also minimize functional loss due to injury. In Chapter 3, Dr Nemoto Mitsuru, and in Chapter 4 Dr Akgun Demir Isil, will introduce the latest developments in optimal wound treatment in severe trauma.

In Chapter 5, we discuss how amputee patients must depend on an artificial leg or arm. It is not easy to find equipment that fits well. Dr Jahmani Rami explains the overgrowth of the stump, which is particularly problematic in cases of amputation in children.

Fortunately, the Paralympic Games will be held in Tokyo in 2020, when this book is published, and we will see many athletes who overcame limb amputation handicaps. I hope this book will help physicians dealing with limb illness and trauma, and all amputee patients.

Masaki Fujioka M.D. Ph.D.
Clinical Professor in the Department of Plastic and Reconstructive Surgery,
Nagasaki University

Director of the Functional Form Research Section, Division of Functional Reconstructive Surgery, and Director of the Department of Plastic and Reconstructive Surgery, National Hospital Organization Nagasaki Medical Center, Ohmura City, Japan

Chapter 1

Introductory Chapter: General Remarks Regarding Limb Amputations

Masaki Fujioka

1. Introduction

Developments of microsurgical techniques allows reimplantation in patients with severed hands, legs, and fingers (**Figures 1** and **2**). And flap transfer techniques have also allowed reconstruction of bone and soft tissue defects in the extremities following malignant neoplasm resection and severe open fractures (**Figures 3** and **4**) [1].

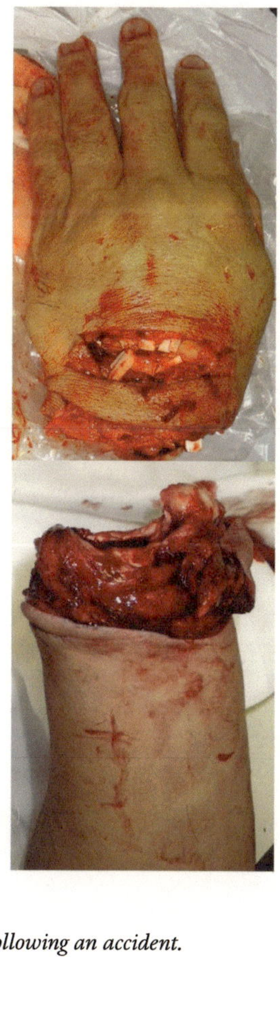

Figure 1.
The photograph shows a severed hand following an accident.

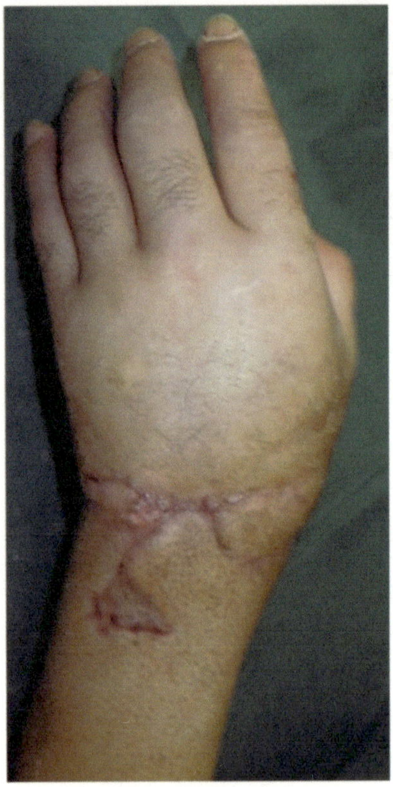

Figure 2.
The photograph shows re-plantation of the severed hand.

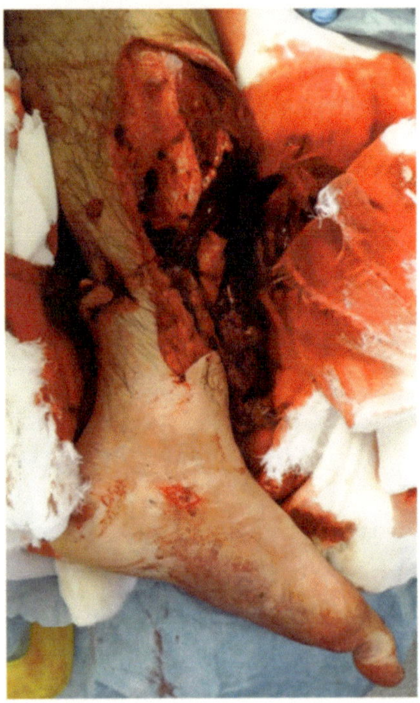

Figure 3.
The photograph shows a Gustilo-Anderson IIIC bone-exposing fracture of the left fibula and tibia with severe abrasion of the skin and muscles.

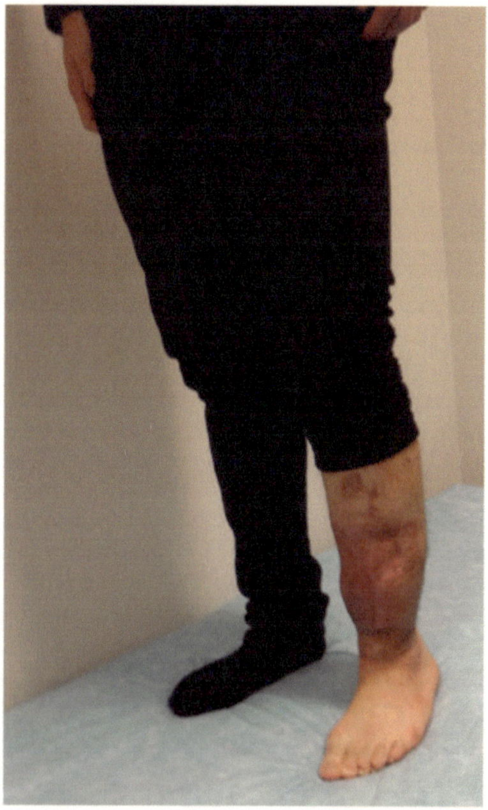

Figure 4.
The patient could walk 1-year after surgery.

As result, previously non-salvageable limbs have been salvaged. However, there are many patients who require limb amputation. Circumstances of limb amputation may vary, including war wound, infections and animal bites, and traffic accidents and various diseases [2, 3].

In this chapter, I describe general remarks regarding limb amputations, which may help to better understand the following chapters.

2. Types and incidence of amputation.

Although the term "amputation" is usually used for the removal of a limb, the removal of other prominent parts of the body, such as the ear, nose, breast, and penis, is also called amputation [4, 5]. However, the population of limb amputees is largest, and an estimated 1.6 million persons were living with the loss of a limb in the USA in the year 2005 [6]. Males are more likely to require limb amputation (a male to female ratio of 1.6–3.9:1), because males are more outgoing and are more prone to trauma, and peripheral artery disease [7]. Lower limb amputation is six–seven times more frequent than upper limbs one [8].

3. Causes

Before 2004, trauma accounted for most amputations in the majority of hospitals, followed by malignancies [9]. Although trauma is still the most predominant indication for amputation in developing countries, peripheral arterial disease with or without diabetes mellitus is now the most common cause of amputation in the developed countries [2, 3].

3.1 Peripheral arterial disease

Limb loss is most often due to peripheral arterial disease (54–82%); the estimated increase in the rate of dysvascular amputations was 27%. On the other hand, rates of trauma- and cancer-related amputations both declined by approximately half [10]. Peripheral arterial disease affects the distal vessels and results in occlusion, which is one of the major causes of ulcer development and a risk factor for amputation (**Figure 5**).

These patients often require challenging distal revascularization surgery or angioplasty to avoid limb amputation. Revascularization is the only way to prevent major amputation of an ischemic foot, and the ulcer healing rate after revascularization ranges from 46 to 91% [11].

3.2 Diabetes mellitus

Patients with diabetes are likely to develop infections, because of the alteration of immune defense mechanisms due to the hyperglycemic environment [12]. Furthermore, more than 50% of patients by diabetes mellitus are complicated with peripheral arterial disease [2].

Once a diabetic foot develops infection, it progresses rapidly and requires the removal of all necrotic tissue (**Figure 6**).

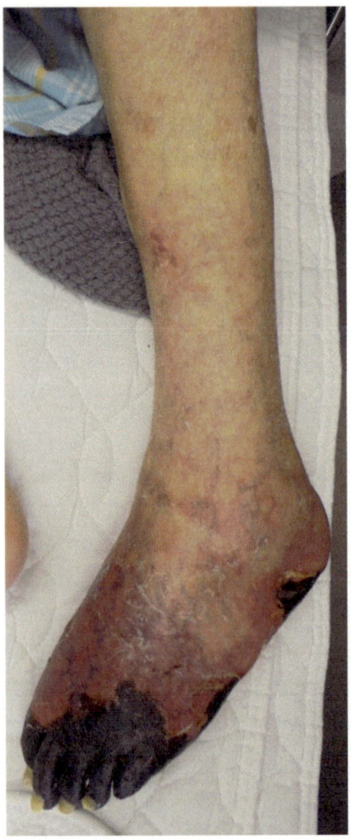

Figure 5.
The photograph shows an ischemic foot due to peripheral arterial disease of the left leg, which required below-knee amputation.

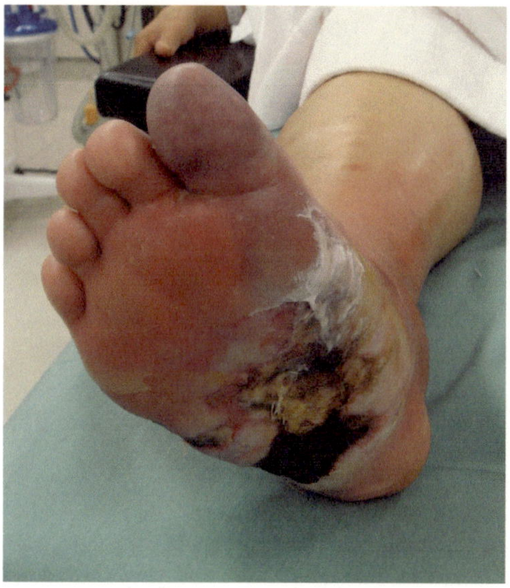

Figure 6.
The photograph shows diabetic gangrene on the right sole, which required transverse tarsal (Chopart) amputations.

These patients are common in developing countries, and extremity amputations associated with diabetes mellitus accounted for most indications (57.0%) in northeast Nigeria [13]. Thus, diabetes prevention, detection, and management should be prioritized in any attempt to reduce the current incidence of amputation [3]

3.3 Infection

Necrotizing fasciitis and myositis are life-threatening infections with associated mortality rates of 10–20% [14]. Especially, *Vibrio vulnificus* and group A streptococci often cause aggressive and fatal gangrene and necrotizing

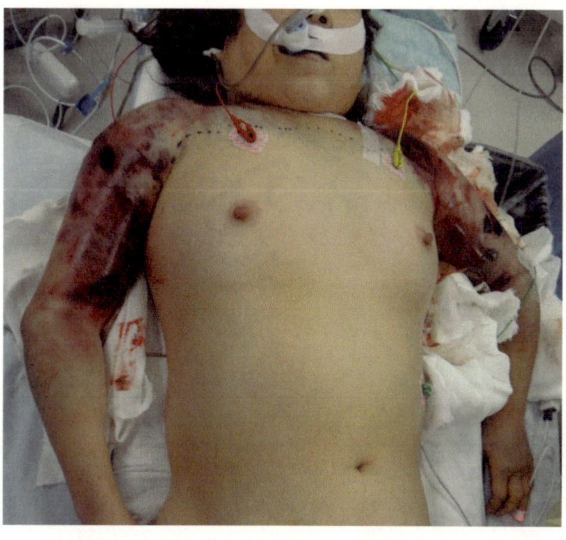

Figure 7.
The photographs show a patient with group a streptococci infection of the bilateral upper lower limbs, which led to streptococcal toxic shock syndrome.

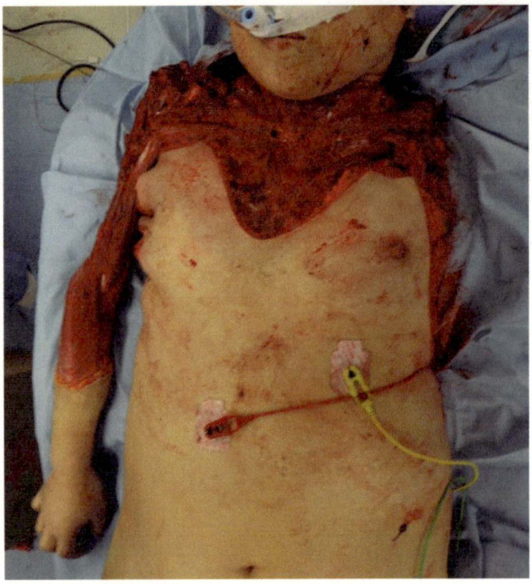

Figure 8.
Intraoperative photographs show immediate amputation of the left arm and the complete removal of the infected skin of the right arm and chest.

myofasciitis, and a reported 23% of patients die of vibrio, and 20–34% die of group A *streptococci* infection [15]. Regarding surgical intervention, early and appropriate debridement to reduce infection is recommended to achieve infection control. Thus, surgical debridement including limb amputation should be considered in the early stage.

Patients with group A *streptococci* infection can develop streptococcal toxic shock syndrome (STSS). When STSS is complicated by myositis, multiple limb amputations should be considered, and the reported mortality rate is 80–100% [16] (**Figures** 7 and **8**).

3.4 Trauma

Treatment of patients with severe injury with vasculopathy of the extremities, such as trauma-related amputation and Gustilo-Anderson type IIIC fracture, is challenging, because it often requires the resurfacing of tissue defects as well as preservation of functional blood flow to distal areas [1]. Previously, patients with these severe limb injuries underwent amputation. Now, most severed limbs can be replanted, and vascular and soft tissue defects can be reconstructed, owing to the development of microsurgical techniques [17]. Therefore, indications for limb amputation due to injuries are now limited.

3.5 Neoplasm

Malignant bone and soft tissue tumors are rare conditions, but a delay in diagnosis or the misinterpretation of data can have limb- and life-threatening consequences. Although a tissue defect following oncologic resection can be reconstructed using a flap transfer technique, hand and leg salvage cannot always be achieved, because radical surgery sometimes requires the removal of important organs such as the bone, arteries, and nerves [17] (**Figure 9**).

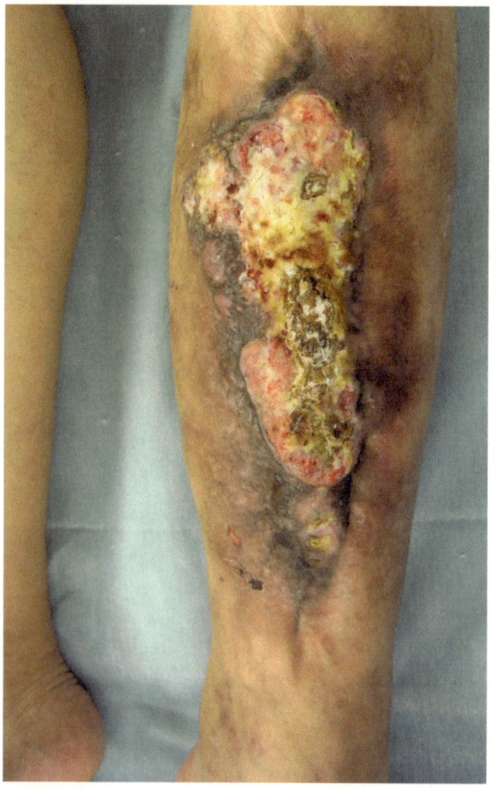

Figure 9.
The photograph shows squamous cell carcinoma on the left leg invading the tibia, which required above-knee amputation.

Conflict of interest statement

There are no conflicts of interest, including financial, consultant, institutional, and other relationships that might lead to a perceived bias.

Financial disclosure and products

There were no external sources of funding in the form of grants supporting the work presented in this manuscript.

Ethical considerations

The procedures followed were in accordance with the ethical standards of our institutional committee on human experimentation and with the Helsinki Declaration of 1975, as revised in 1983.

Patients in our manuscript were additionally informed about the patient's ethical rights by the author and agreed that the patient's illustrative material, including face, could be used for the aim of the medical study and also agreed to the photos being published in a medical journal.

This manuscript has not previously been presented at any meeting. This article is original and has not previously been published.

Author details

Masaki Fujioka
Department of Plastic and Reconstructive Surgery, Clinical Research Center, National Hospital Organization Nagasaki Medical Center, Nagasaki, Japan

*Address all correspondence to: inazmahayato7@gmail.com

References

[1] Fujioka M. Application of free flow-through anterolateral thigh flap for the reconstruction of an extremity soft tissue defect requiring vascularization. In: Flap Surgery. Rijeka: InTech; 2018. pp. 51-76 (Chapter 4)

[2] Yaghi K, Yaghi Y, McDonald AA, Yadegarfar G, Cecil E, Seidl J, et al. Diabetes or war? Incidence of and indications for limb amputation in Lebanon, 2007. Eastern Mediterranean Health Journal. 2012;**18**(12):1178-1186

[3] Sargen MR, Hoffstad O, Margolis DJ. Geographic variation in Medicare spending and mortality for diabetic patients with foot ulcers and amputations. Journal of Diabetes and its Complications. 2013;**27**(2):128-133

[4] Ellis H. Amputation of the breast. Journal of Perioperative Practice. 2015;**25**(1-2):27-28

[5] Falcone M, Garaffa G, Raheem A, Christopher NA, Ralph DJ. Total phallic reconstruction using the radial artery based forearm free flap after traumatic penile amputation. The Journal of Sexual Medicine. 2016;**13**(7):1119-1124

[6] Ziegler-Graham K, MacKenzie EJ, Ephraim PL, Travison TG, Brookmeyer R. Estimating the prevalence of limb loss in the United States: 2005 to 2050. Archives of Physical Medicine and Rehabilitation. 2008;**89**(3):422-429

[7] Roumia M, Aronow HD, Soukas P, Gosch K, Smolderen KG, Spertus JA, et al. Sex differences in disease-specific health status measures in patients with symptomatic peripheral artery disease: Data from the PORTRAIT study. Vascular Medicine. 2017;**22**(2):103-109

[8] Farrokhi S, Perez K, Eskridge S, Clouser M. Major deployment-related amputations of lower and upper limbs, active and reserve components, U.S. Armed Forces, 2001-2017. MSMR. 2018;**25**(7):10-16

[9] Settakorn J, Rangdaeng S, Arpornchayanon O, Lekawanvijit S, Bhoopat L, Attia J. Why were limbs amputated? An evaluation of 216 surgical specimens from Chiang Mai University Hospital, Thailand. Archives of Orthopaedic and Trauma Surgery. 2005;**125**(10):701-705

[10] Dillingham TR, Pezzin LE, MacKenzie EJ. Limb amputation and limb deficiency: Epidemiology and recent trends in the United States. Southern Medical Journal. 2002;**95**(8):875-883

[11] Vouillarmet J, Bourron O, Gaudric J, Lermusiaux P, Millon A, Hartemann A. Lower-extremity arterial revascularization: Is there any evidence for diabetic foot ulcer-healing? Diabetes & Metabolism. 2016;**42**(1):4-15

[12] Mustăţea P, Bugă C, Doran H, Mihalache O, Bobîrcă FT, Georgescu DE, et al. Soft tissue infections in diabetic patients. Chirurgia (Bucur). 2018;**113**(5):651-667

[13] Dabkana TM, Nyaku FT, Bwala ST. Current indications for extremity amputations in Maiduguri, north-East Nigeria: A 6-year retrospective review. Annals of African Medicine. 2018;**17**(1):22-25

[14] Fujioka M, Nishimura G, Miyazato O, et al. Necrotizing fasciitis and myositis that originated from gastrointestinal bacterial infection: Two fatel cases. Scandinavian Journal of Plastic and Reconstructive Surgery and Hand Surgery. 2003;**37**:239-242

[15] Kaul R, McGeer A, Low DE, Green K, Schwartz B. Population-based surveillance for group A streptococcal necrotizing fasciitis: Clinical features,

prognostic indicators, and microbiologic analysis of seventy-seven cases. Ontario Group A Streptococcal Study. American Journal of Medicine. 1997;**103**(1):18-24

[16] Saijo H, Fujioka M, Hayashida K, Murakami C. A fatal case of streptococcal toxic shock syndrome by group A *streptococcus* despite of undergoing immediate three extremities amputation. Japanese Journal of Plastic & Reconstructive Surgery. 2013;**56**:667-672

[17] Saint-Cyr M, Langstein HN. Reconstruction of the hand and upper extremity after tumor resection. Journal of Surgical Oncology. 2006;**94**:490-503

Chapter 2

A Retrospective Analysis of Amputation Risk Due to Diabetic Foot and Angioplasty and Free Flap Transfer to Reduce Major Amputation

Masaki Fujioka

Abstract

Foot ulceration in persons with diabetes is the most frequent precursor to amputation, which impairs their activities. The aim of this chapter is to describe factors that lead to amputation of a diabetic foot, and propose a management strategy to prevent major amputation. I analyzed 233 patients who were admitted at the National Nagasaki Medical Center between 2008 and 2017 with foot ulcer and/or infection. We divided them into two groups: 152 patients with diabetes mellitus (DM) and 81 without DM. We analyzed their laboratory data, and evaluated the wound severity, complications of peripheral artery disease (PAD) and renal failure, and infection. Patients with DM ulcer were significantly more likely to receive amputation. Patients with DM were significantly more likely to develop infection, and tended to undergo emergency debridement. Among the patients with DM, the amputation group (85) showed significantly higher levels of CRP and WBC, and was more likely to develop infection, PAD, and renal failure. My results suggest that risk factors leading to leg amputation are severe infection and reduction of arterial blood flow. Early debridement to reduce infectious inflammation and angioplasty following free flap transfer are recommended to preserve legs.

Keywords: diabetic foot, diabetic gangrene, leg amputation, angioplasty, free flap transfer

1. Introduction

In the past four decades, over 42–56% of major lower extremity amputations in the United States and Western European countries have been due to diabetes mellitus (DM) [1–4]. The relative risk of major leg amputations for diabetes ranges from 5.1 to 31.5 times in comparison with that of nondiabetic populations [5, 6]. Extensive efforts have been made to improve the treatment of diabetes in regard to glycemic control and the prevention of diabetic complications, and foot ulcer treatments have improved for diabetic patients [7, 8]. Before 2004, trauma accounted for most amputations in the majority of hospitals, followed by malignancies [9]. However, the most common cause of amputation at present is diabetes mellitus [10, 11].

Amputation is the most appropriate therapy for an ischemic or infected limb, but the level at which to amputate is often difficult to determine. Patients who undergo only toe or trans-metatarsal amputation can walk on their own feet; however, those with major amputation require an artificial leg or a cane, which impairs their activities [12, 13]. The aim of this chapter is to describe factors that lead to amputation of a diabetic foot and propose a management strategy to prevent major amputation.

2. Materials and methods

A retrospective descriptive study including 152 diabetic patients among 233 patients with leg ulcers who were treated in our medical center was carried out between January 2008 and December 2017. All patients had been diagnosed with type II diabetes. Diabetic foot ulcers represent more than 65 percent of all leg ulcers.

To clarify the clinical characteristics of the diabetic foot, a comparison of foot ulcer patients with and without diabetes mellitus is conducted first, risk factors leading to amputation in cases of diabetic foot ulcer and "major" amputation in cases of diabetic foot are discussed, and a recommended strategy to avoid major leg amputation is presented.

Statistical analysis was performed using the *Wilcoxon* signed-rank *test and* chi-square test. The *value* of $p < 0.05$ was determined as *significant*.

The ethical committee of our medical center approved this study.

3. Results

3.1 Comparison of foot ulcer patients with and without diabetes mellitus

Profiles of foot ulcer patients with and without diabetes mellitus are shown in **Table 1**. Of the 233 patients with a foot ulcer, 63% (147) were men, and 37% (86) were women. Of course, levels of HbA1C and blood sugar in the diabetic foot group were significantly higher than those in the nondiabetic foot group, and men were more likely to develop leg ulcers in the diabetic patient group. There were no significant differences in CRP, WBC, serum albumin, or hemoglobin between the groups.

The severity of leg ulcers at discovery in patients with and without diabetes mellitus is shown in **Table 2**. In the groups, the ulcer stage based on the Wagner classification showed similar tendencies. About 80% of the diabetic foot group developed infection, being a significantly higher rate than in the nondiabetic foot. Methicillin-resistant *Staphylococcus aureus* (MRSA), methicillin-susceptible *Staphylococcus aureus* (MSSA), and *Streptococcus* were ranked high and accounted for over three-quarters of infections in both groups (**Figure 1**).

Because patients with diabetes are likely to develop severe infection, more than 50% of foot ulcer patients with diabetes required immediate debridement surgery, being a significantly higher rate than in the nondiabetic foot group (25%) (**Figure 2**).

The frequencies of peripheral artery disease in foot ulcer patients with and without diabetes were 38.2 and 34.6%, respectively. There were no significant differences between the groups.

The frequencies of hemodialysis in patients with and without diabetes were 7.2 and 6.2%, respectively. There were no significant differences between the groups.

DOI: http://dx.doi.org/10.5772/intechopen.88351

	Diabetic foot ulcer (152)	Non-diabetic foot ulcer (81)	P-value
Male/Female	104/48	43/38	P<0.05*
Age	66.3±14.0	65.0±17.1	0.11
Hb A1C (%)	8.7±2.6	5.4±0.8	p<0.001
Blood Sugar (mg/L)	258.5±127.8	119.5±6.4	p<0.001
CRP (mg/L)	128.2±90.6	110.9±89.8	0.24
WBC (×10⁹/L)	12.1±7.1	11.5±5.5	0.83
S-Albumin (g/dL)	2.9±0.8	3.3±1.2	0.05
Hemoglobin (g/dL)	10.8±2.5	11.0±2.1	0.98
Hospitalization period (days)	39.6±36.6	32.1±32.6	0.45

(Wilcoxon rank sum test *: Chi-squared test)

Table 1.
Profile of foot ulcer patients with and without diabetes mellitus.

Wagner Classification	Diabetic foot ulcer (152)	Non-diabetic foot ulcer(81)	P-value Chi-squared test
1 (superficial ulcer)	14(9.2%)	9(11.1%)	P>0.05
2 (deep ulcer)	24(15.8%)	21(25.9%)	P>0.05
3 (osteomyelitis or abscess)	47(31.0%)	19(23.5%)	P>0.05
4 (forefoot gangrene)	25(16.4%)	13(16.0%)	P>0.05
5 (whole foot gangrene)	42(27.6%)	19(23.4%)	P>0.05

Table 2.
Severity of leg ulcers at discovery in patients with and without diabetes mellitus.

The frequencies of amputation in foot ulcer patients with and without diabetes were 53.9 and 34.6%, respectively. More than half of the patients with diabetes underwent amputation surgery, being a significantly higher rate than that in the nondiabetic foot group (**Figure 3**).

3.2 Comparison of foot ulcer patients with and without diabetes mellitus

We evaluated 85 amputated legs in 152 diabetic foot patients. Sixty-eight percent (104) of the patients were men, and 32% (48) were women. Profiles of diabetic patients with/without leg amputation are shown in **Table 3**.

Men were more likely to require amputation. CRP and WBC were significantly higher, and serum albumin was significantly lower in the major amputation group, suggesting that severe infection and malnutrition are risk factors for major leg amputation in diabetic foot patients.

	Diabetic foot ulcer (152)	Non-diabetic foot ulcer (81)	P-value
Infection	121 (79.6%)	49 (53.3%)	<0.001*

*: Chi-squared test)

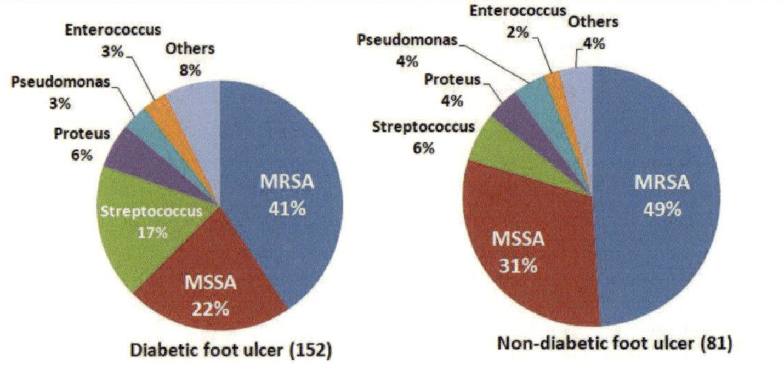

Figure 1.
Infection of leg ulcers at discovery in patients with and without diabetes mellitus (MRSA, methicillin-resistant Staphylococcus aureus; MSSA, methicillin-susceptible Staphylococcus aureus).

	Diabetic foot ulcer(152)	Non-diabetic foot ulcer(81)	P value
Immediate surgery	79(52.0%)	20 (25.0%)	<0.001*

*: Chi-squared test)

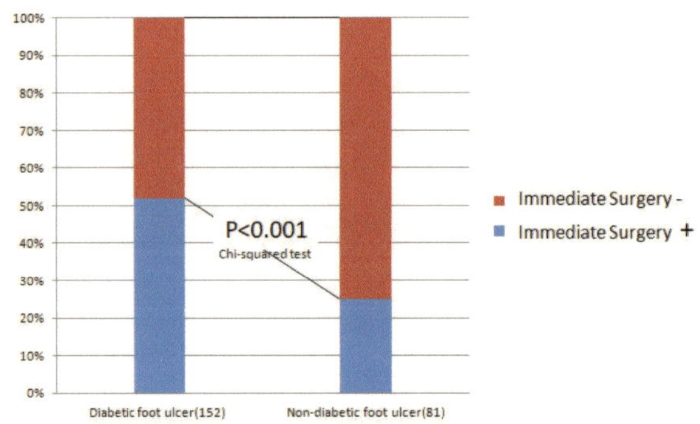

Figure 2.
The frequency of foot ulcer patients with and without diabetes, who required immediate debridement surgery.

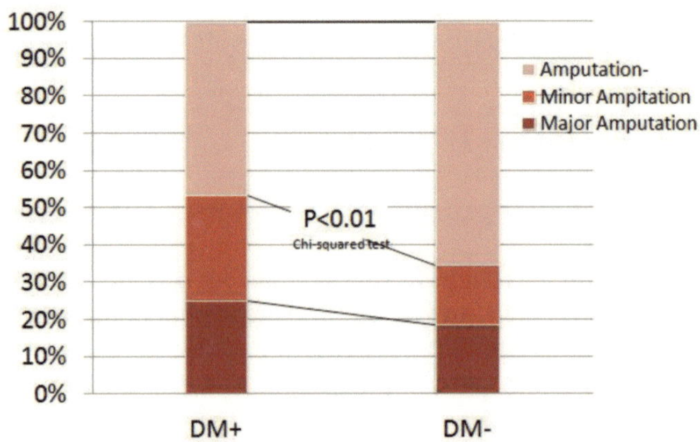

Figure 3.
The frequency of amputation in foot ulcer patients with and without diabetes.

	Amputation+ (85)	Amputation- (67)	P-value
Male/Female	61/24	43/24	<0.05*
Age	65.0±17.1	66.3±14.0	0.35
Hb A1C (%)	8.5±2.2	8.8±2.7	0.67
Blood Sugar (mg/L)	251.2±122.6	262.1±129.5	0.90
CRP (mg/L)	202.0±93.1	115.6±89.9	0.001
WBC ($\times 10^9$/L)	17.1±8.8	10.9±6.1	0.017
S-Albumin (g/dL)	2.5±0.7	3.0±0.8	0.016
Hemoglobin (g/dL)	10.5±2.2	11.0±2.6	0.10

(Wilcoxon rank sum test *: Chi-squared test)

Table 3.
Profiles of diabetic patients with and without leg amputation.

Sixty-nine (82%) of 85 amputees and 36 (57.6%) of 67 non-amputees with diabetes developed infection, showing a significant difference between the groups. More than half of amputated and only 17.9% of non-amputated patients with diabetes were complicated by peripheral artery disease, showing a significant difference between the groups (**Figure 4**). Furthermore, the frequency of hemodialysis in amputated patients (11.8%) was also significantly higher than that in non-amputated patients (1.5%) (**Figure 5**).

3.3 Comparison of diabetic foot ulcer patients who underwent major and minor leg amputation

Of the 85 amputees with diabetes, 44 patients underwent minor amputation, and 38 received major amputation. Seventy-one percent (58) were men and 29% (24) were women. Profiles of diabetic patients with/without leg amputation are shown in **Table 4**. Men were more likely to require major amputation. CRP and WBC were significantly higher, and serum albumin was significantly lower in the

	Diabetic foot ulcer(152)	Non-diabetic foot ulcer(81)	P value Chi-squared test
Peripheral Artery Disease	58(38.2%)	28 (34.6%)	>0.05*

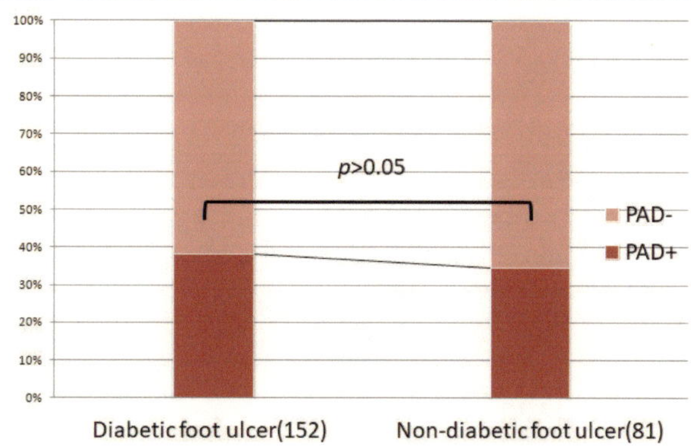

Figure 4.
The frequency of amputation in diabetic foot ulcer patients with and without peripheral artery disease.

	Diabetic foot ulcer(152)	Non-diabetic foot ulcer(81)	P value Chi-squared test
Hemodialysis(HD)	11(7.2%)	5 (6.2%)	>0.05*

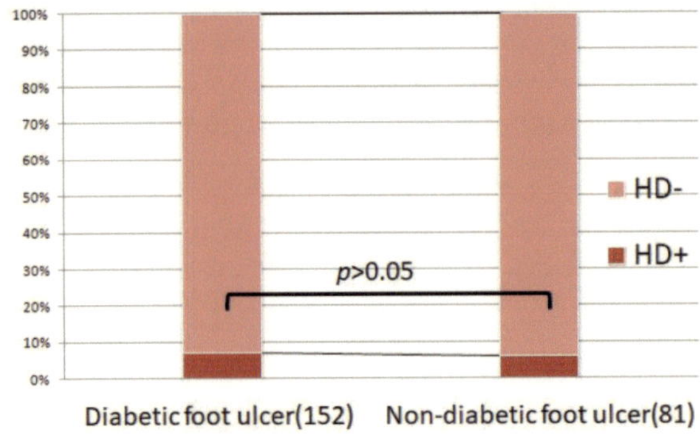

Figure 5.
The frequency of amputation in diabetic foot ulcer patients with and without hemodialysis.

	Major Amputation+ (38)	Minor Amputation- (44)	P-value
Male/Female	31/7	27/17	<0.05*
Age	68.7.0±14.4	65.9±12.5	0.31
Hb A1C (%)	8.5±2.2	9.2±3.2	0.18
Blood Sugar (mg/L)	250.2±121.1	269.6±145.1	0.61
CRP (mg/L)	200.8±92.3	85.4±58.6	<0.001
WBC (× 10^9/L)	17.0±8.7	9.0±4.8	<0.001
S-Albumin (g/dL)	2.5±0.7	3.1±0.7	0.002
Hemoglobin (g/dL)	10.4±2.2	10.6±2.4	0.50

(Wilcoxon rank sum test *: Chi-squared test)

Table 4.
Profiles of diabetic patients who underwent major and minor leg amputation.

major amputation group, suggesting that severe infection and malnutrition are risk factors for major leg amputation in diabetic foot patients.

4. Risk factors leading to leg amputation and strategy to prevent major amputation

Diabetic foot ulcers sometimes lead to minor or major amputation, with a high impact on patients' life and its quality [14]. Our results suggest that risk factors for leg amputation in diabetic foot patients include male, complication of severe infection, complication of peripheral artery disease, complication of hemodialysis, and malnutrition.

4.1 Improvement of malnutrition

The importance of nutritional support in patients with wounds has been examined. Malnourished patients showed not only a higher frequency of impaired wound healing but also an increased risk of postoperative cardiopulmonary and septic complications [15, 16]. Malnutrition cannot be improved in a short time after developing foot ulcers. Thus, patients requiring surgical treatment should also receive supplemental nourishment in the perioperative period [17]. Luo et al. suggested that the geriatric nutritional risk index was a reliable and effective predictive marker of patients' amputation-free survival, and it could identify patients early with a high risk of amputation [18]. Appropriate blood sugar control and nutritional support are required for diabetic patients to prevent leg amputation. Malnutrition usually occurs in critical limb ischemia patients as well, because of a lack of appetite and sleeplessness due to chronic pain. These patients with peripheral artery disease also require pain control and nutritional support services [18].

4.2 Foot care for patients undergoing hemodialysis

The number of patients requiring hemodialysis has been growing because obesity-related renal diseases such as diabetes mellitus are increasing [19, 20]. Diabetic patients with renal failure had high risks of foot ulceration and lower limb complications [21]. Regarding cutaneous infection, Bencini et al. reported that the incidence of fungal infection in patients undergoing hemodialysis was 67% [22]. Because chronic renal failure patients exhibit impaired cellular immunity due to a decreased T-lymphocyte cell count, this could explain the increased prevalence of fungal infections [23]· Thus, difficulty healing wounds is a frequent problem in patients on hemodialysis [24]. Amputations of limbs are sometimes performed for these complex ulcers, because when patients receiving hemodialysis develop aggressive life-threatening infections such as sepsis, immediate surgical debridement is required in order to salvage the blood access line and save lives [25]. Fujioka reported that 13 of 17 wounds required immediate surgery, including amputation and debridement in patients with DM, while only 1 of 13 required immediate surgery in patients without DM [26].

Poor management of foot ulcers in patients receiving hemodialysis leads to prolonged ulceration, gangrene, amputation, depression, and death [27].

Marn et al. investigated the association between the implementation of a routine foot check program in diabetic incident hemodialysis patients and concluded that monthly foot checks are associated with a reduction of major lower limb amputations [28]. All patients on hemodialysis should be considered as being at high risk of developing foot complications and undergo foot checks frequently. If infection is suspected, antibiotics should be administered through the dialysis line immediately during dialysis.

4.3 Infection control

Diabetic foot infection is a common diabetic complication, which results in lower limb amputation if not treated properly. Patients with diabetes are likely to develop infections, because of the alteration of immune defense mechanisms such as a change in the neutrophil function, suppression of the antioxidant system, and modified humoral activity due to the hyperglycemic environment [29].

Once a diabetic foot develops infection, it progresses rapidly and requires the removal of all necrotizing tissue involving the bone, tendons, and skin (**Figure 6**).

If the toe infection progresses and spreads widely, the patient may have to undergo major amputation (**Figures 7a** and **b**). Thus, early and appropriate debridement to reduce infection is important.

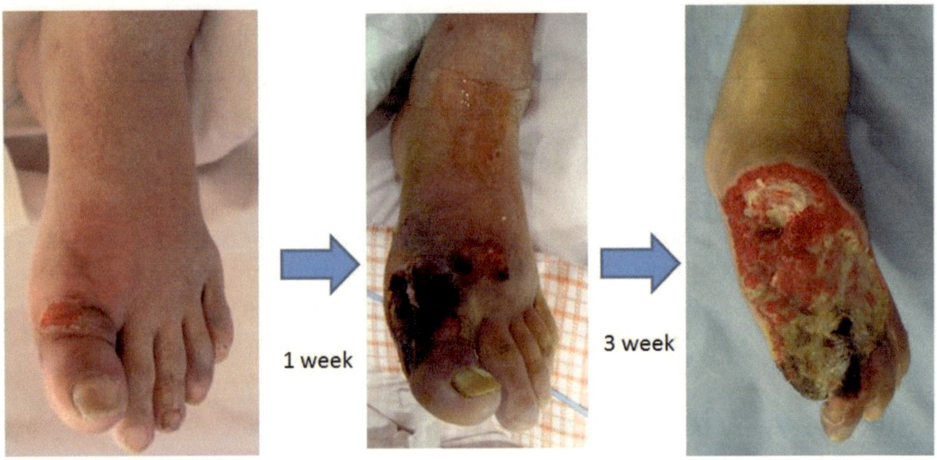

Figure 6.
A view of progressing diabetic infection in the big toe, which aggravated rapidly and required the removal of toes and metatarsal bones within 3 weeks.

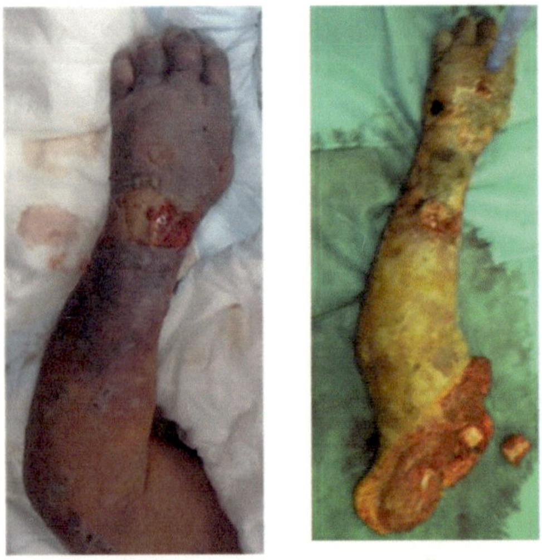

Figure 7.
(a) A view of necrotizing fasciitis in the left forearm at the first examination, which progressed rapidly to the upper arm, and the patient developed septic shock in 2 days. (b) Amputation of the infected hand at the upper arm was immediately performed to control the aggressive infection.

4.3.1 Antibiotic treatment

Soft tissue infections in diabetic patients require multidisciplinary treatment including rapid surgical intervention, antibiotic treatment, and hyperbaric oxygen therapy to restrict the growth of pathogens [30–32]. Antibiotic therapy should be instituted immediately. The initial antibiotic should act on aerobic Gram-positive and Gram-negative bacteria but also on anaerobic bacteria. Systemic antibiotics have been demonstrated in many trials to be effective in treating acute diabetic foot infections. Tchero et al. performed a systematic review to assess the clinical efficacy of antibiotic regimens in the treatment of diabetic foot infections and concluded that piperacillin/tazobactam should be recommended for severe infections and the adjuvant use of topical agents with systemic antibiotics improved the outcomes compared with systemic antibiotics alone [33]. Mustățea et al. suggested that an initial combination of third-generation cephalosporin, quinolone, and metronidazole was initially administered. After germ identification, antibiotic therapy was administered according to the antibiogram [29]. Cellulitis, which shows inflammation and infection of the skin and subcutaneous tissue, can be treated with systemic Gram-positive bactericidal antibiotics only. However, if deep tissue infection, especially osteomyelitis, is suspected, removal of the infected bone and soft tissue, followed by 2–4 weeks of antibiotics, is required [30].

4.3.2 Surgical debridement

Regarding surgical intervention, early and appropriate debridement to reduce infection is recommended to achieve infection control (**Figure 8**).

If the infection invades deeper to the tendon, the lesions can often be extended and spread upward rapidly along the tendon tract, which can lead to systematic sepsis and require immediate limb amputation (**Figure 9a** and **b**). As the infection developing in the diabetic patients' limbs progresses rapidly, physicians must decide on whether to carry out debridement before the infected lesion spreads upward.

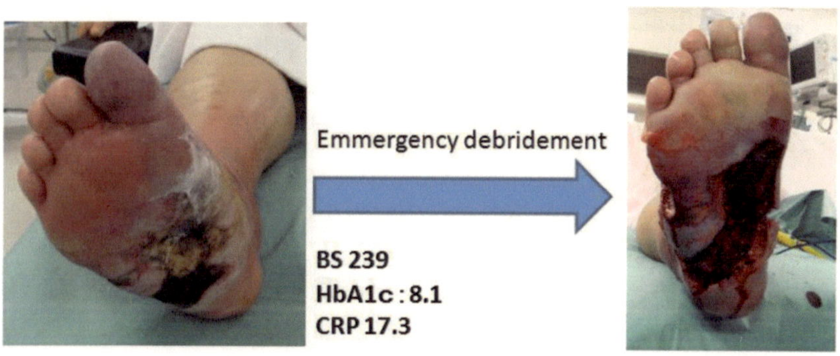

Figure 8.
Views of debridement for necrotizing fasciitis in the diabetic patient's right sole. All necrotizing, contaminated tissue was removed immediately.

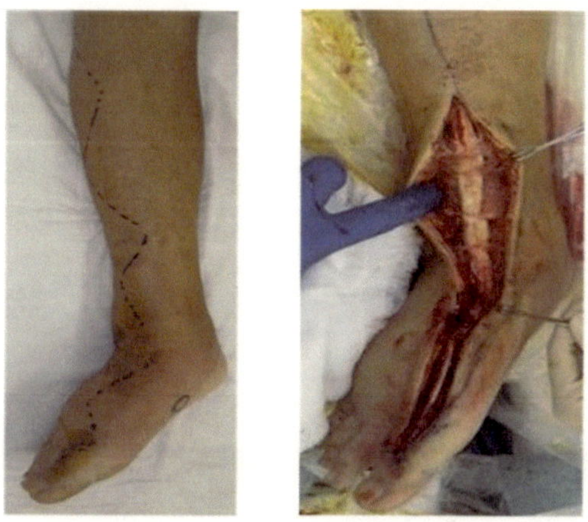

a b

Figure 9.
(a) A view of necrotizing fasciitis in the right big toe, which spreads upward rapidly.
(b) Intraoperative view showing the contaminated lesion extending along the extensor tendon tract.

Case presentations

Case 1. A 51-year-old man developed diabetic foot gangrene with osteomyelitis of the fifth toe, which had progressed for 2 weeks (**Figure 10a**). The patient underwent fourth and fifth toe amputation immediately, and cleansing to reduce infection was performed for 2 weeks (**Figure 10b**). As abundant granulation tissue developed on the wound surface, he underwent free skin grafting (**Figure 10c**). The wound had completely resurfaced by 1 month after skin grafting, and the patient could walk without a cane (**Figure 10d**).

4.3.3 Angioplasty for an ischemic foot

Peripheral artery disease (PAD) is observed in up to 50% of patients with a diabetic foot ulcer, and the presence of PAD is an important consideration in their management [34]. PAD affects the distal vessels and results in occlusion, which is one of the major causes of ulcer development and an increased risk of amputation. The treatment for these patients often requires challenging distal revascularization surgery or angioplasty to prevent limb amputation [35]. Revascularization is commonly performed in patients with critical limb ischemia and a diabetic foot ulcer, and the ulcer-healing rate after revascularization ranges from 46 to 91% [36]. Hinchliffe et al. reviewed the effectiveness of revascularization of the ulcerated foot in patients with diabetes and PAD 1 year after surgery and reported that limb salvage rates showed a median of 85% following open surgery, and more than 60% of ulcers had healed following revascularization. They concluded that revascularization improved rates of limb salvage compared with the results of conservatively treated patients [34].

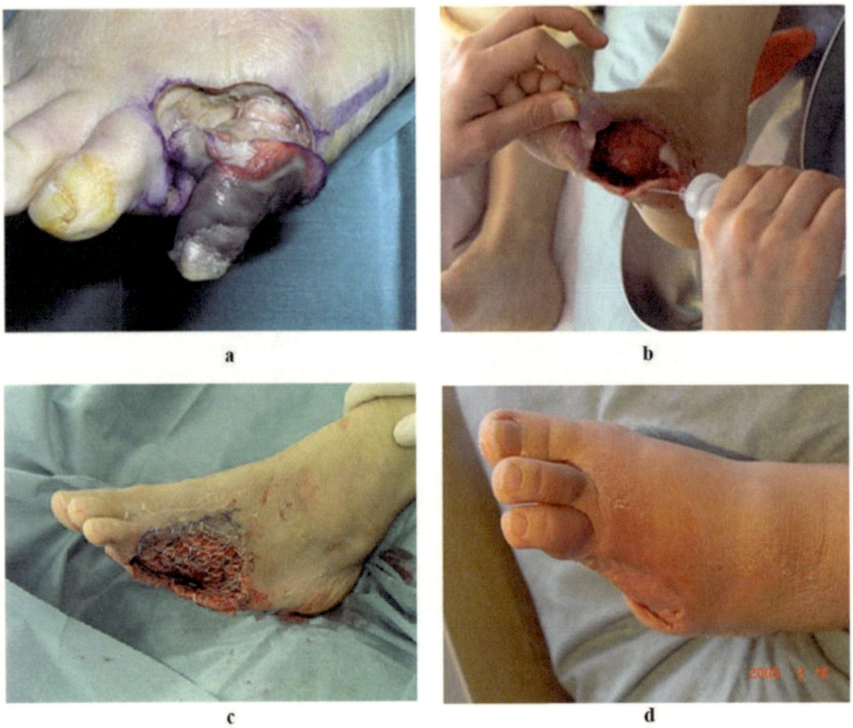

Figure 10.
(a) Case 1. A view of diabetic foot gangrene with osteomyelitis of the fifth toe. (b) After fourth and fifth toe amputation, cleansing was performed for 2 weeks. (c) Intraoperative view showing free skin grafting on the wound. (d) A view of the foot 1 month after surgery showing favorable coverage of the wound.

Case presentations

Case 2. A 67-year-old man developed a diabetic foot ulcer of the right heel, which had progressed for 2 months (**Figure 11a**). His posterior tibial artery was not palpable. Enhanced computed tomography (CT) showed that circulation of his right lower leg was poor, with an ankle brachial pressure index (ABI) of only 0.53, which suggested that his leg ulcer might not heel spontaneously. We fashioned femoral-popliteal artery (FP) bypass to increase distal blood flow, and ABI improved to 0.83(**Figure 11b**). As the patient's foot received sufficient flow, he could safely undergo resurfacing surgery using a reversed sural flap successfully and could walk 3 months after surgery (**Figure 11c–f**).

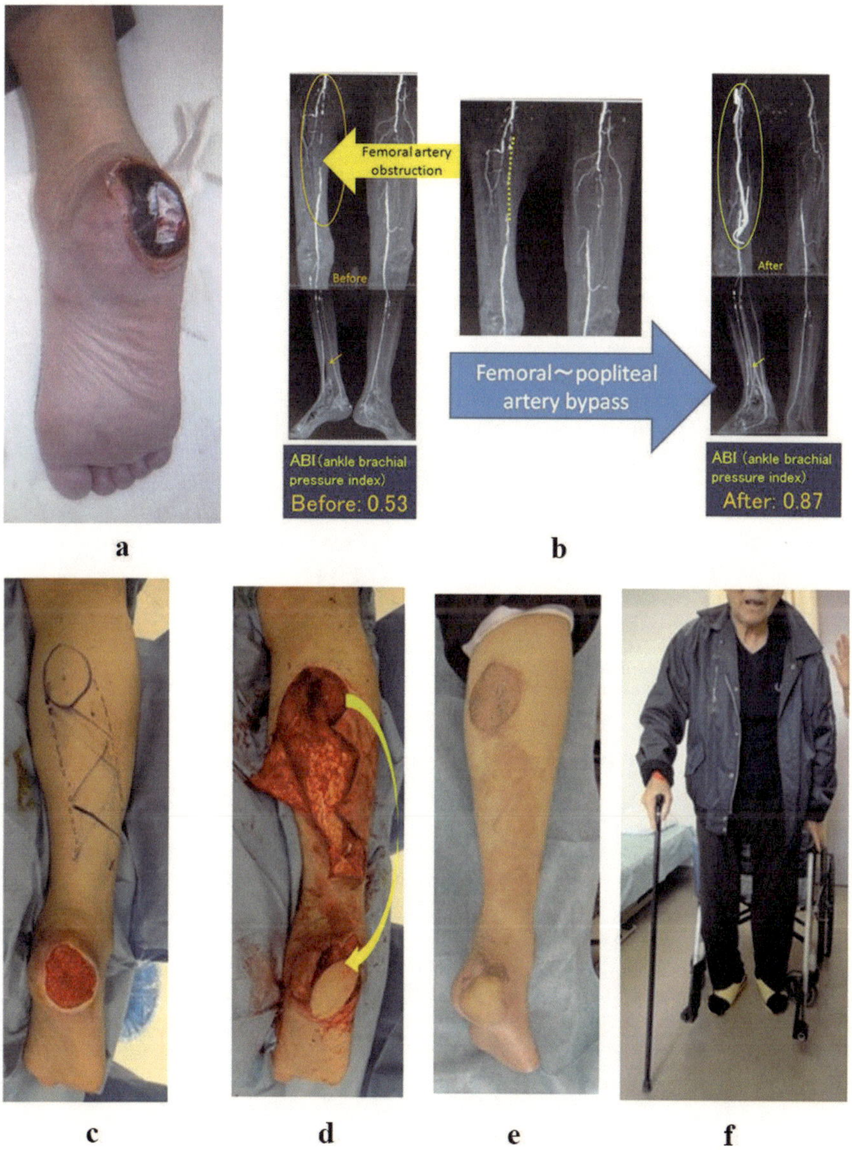

Figure 11.
(a) Case 2. A view of a diabetic foot ulcer of the right heel. (b) Enhanced computed tomography scan image showing the poor circulation of the patient's right lower leg due to obstruction of the right femoral artery (circles). After fashioning the femoral-popliteal artery bypass, increased distal blood flow was seen (small arrows). (c) Intraoperative view showing the debrided heel ulcer and design of the reversed sural flap. (d) Intraoperative view of heel reconstruction showing the transferred reversed sural flap. (e) A view of the reconstructed heel 3 months after surgery revealed favorable coverage of the wound. (f) The patient could walk 3 months after surgery.

Case 3. A 60-year-old man developed a diabetic foot ulcer and osteomyelitis of the calcaneus (**Figure 12a**). Following the removal of a sequester, he underwent FP bypass angioplasty, and ABI improved from 0.67 to 1.01 (**Figure 12b**). The bone-exposing wound was resurfaced using a free superficial circumflex iliac perforator (SCIP) flap (**Figure 12c–e**). One year after the surgery, good circulation had been achieved without infection or ulcer relapse (**Figure 12f**).

4.3.4 Advantages of resurfacing the amputation stump with a free flap

Standard stump plasty requires shortening of the remaining fine and vivid bone end to resurface the bone-exposing amputation stump (**Figure 13a** and **b**).

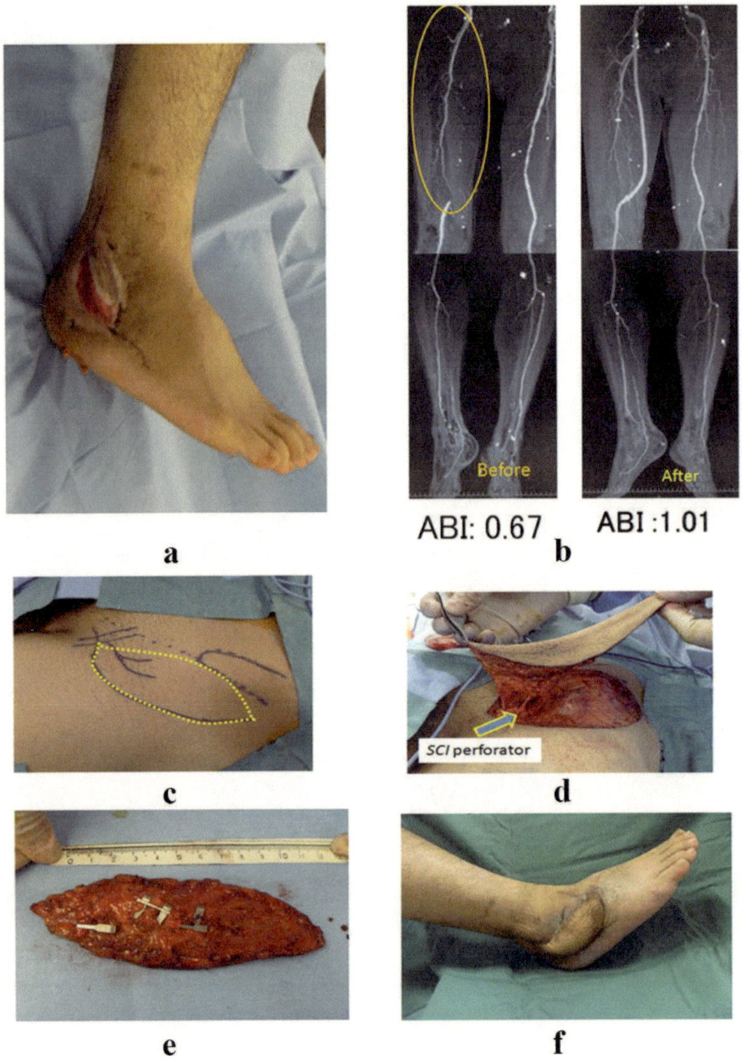

Figure 12.
(a) Case 3. A view of a diabetic foot ulcer and osteomyelitis of the calcaneus. (b) Enhanced computed tomography scan image showing poor circulation of the patient's right lower leg due to obstruction of right femoral artery (circle). After fashioning the femoral-popliteal artery bypass, increased distal blood flow was seen. (c) Intraoperative view showing the design of a free superficial circumflex iliac perforator flap. (d) Intraoperative view of the elevated SCIP flap. The arrow indicates the perforator of superficial circumflex iliac vessels. (e) Intraoperative view of the harvested SCIP flap. (f) A view of the reconstructed foot 1 year after surgery showing favorable coverage of the wound.

On the other hand, free flap transfer enables surgeons to maintain the bone length, which is a potential advantage, especially when amputation is performed at the trans-metatarsal lesion (**Figure 14a–c**).

This is because Chopart or transtibial amputation results in more debilitating functional outcomes than transmetatarsal amputation. Furthermore, transmetatarsal amputation preserves maximal foot length, allowing patients to achieve a better quality of life [37, 38].

Regarding the flap choice, the ideal flap is thought to be a good vascularized skin paddle with the same thickness and width as the wound and requiring a single-stage operation [39]. Perforator flaps are defined as flaps consisting of skin and/or subcutaneous fat, with a blood supply from isolated perforating vessels of a stem artery [40]. The development of perforator flaps has increased the number of potential donor sites because a flap can be supplied by any musculocutaneous perforator, and donor-site morbidity can be reduced [41, 42]. Furthermore, the advantage of this skin flap is that it is less invasive, so that the operation can be performed under local anesthesia if the wound is small.

Case presentation

Case 4. A 32-year-old man developed a diabetic foot ulcer on the step (**Figure 15a**). Following debridement, he underwent resurfacing surgery using a free superficial circumflex Iliac artery perforator flap (**Figure 12b** and **c**). As free SCIP flap transfer is less invasive, the operation can be performed under local anesthesia (**Figure 15d**). One year after the surgery, good circulation had been achieved without infection or ulcer relapse (**Figure 15e**).

The SCIP flap is recommended because it minimizes sacrifice at the donor site, causing no damage to the main vessels or muscles beneath the flap. The only disadvantage is that the pedicle vessel is sometimes short when a suitable recipient vessel cannot

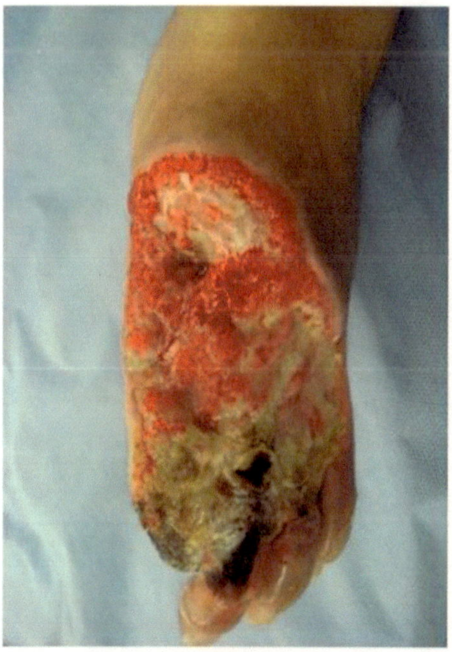
(a)

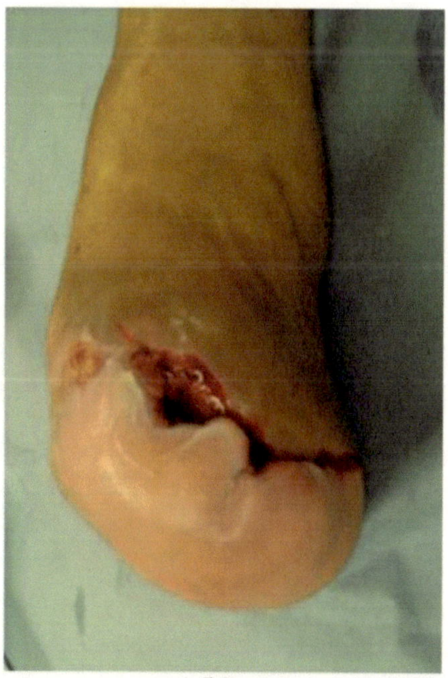
(b)

Figure 13.
(a) A view of diabetic gangrene extending the first and second metatarsal bones. After removal of the necrotic bone, the navicular was exposed. (b) Intraoperative view of Chopart amputation followed by resurfacing with a local flap of the sole.

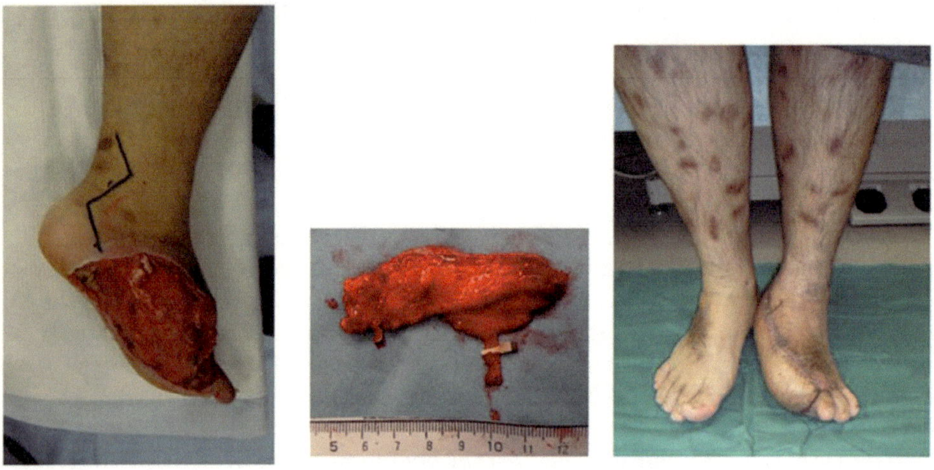

Figure 14.
(a) A view of a diabetic foot ulcer with osteomyelitis of the first and second metatarsal bones. (b) Intraoperative view of the harvested anterolateral thigh (ALT) flap. (c) A view of the reconstructed foot using a free ALT flap 1 year after surgery, showing favorable coverage, and the patient could walk without a cane.

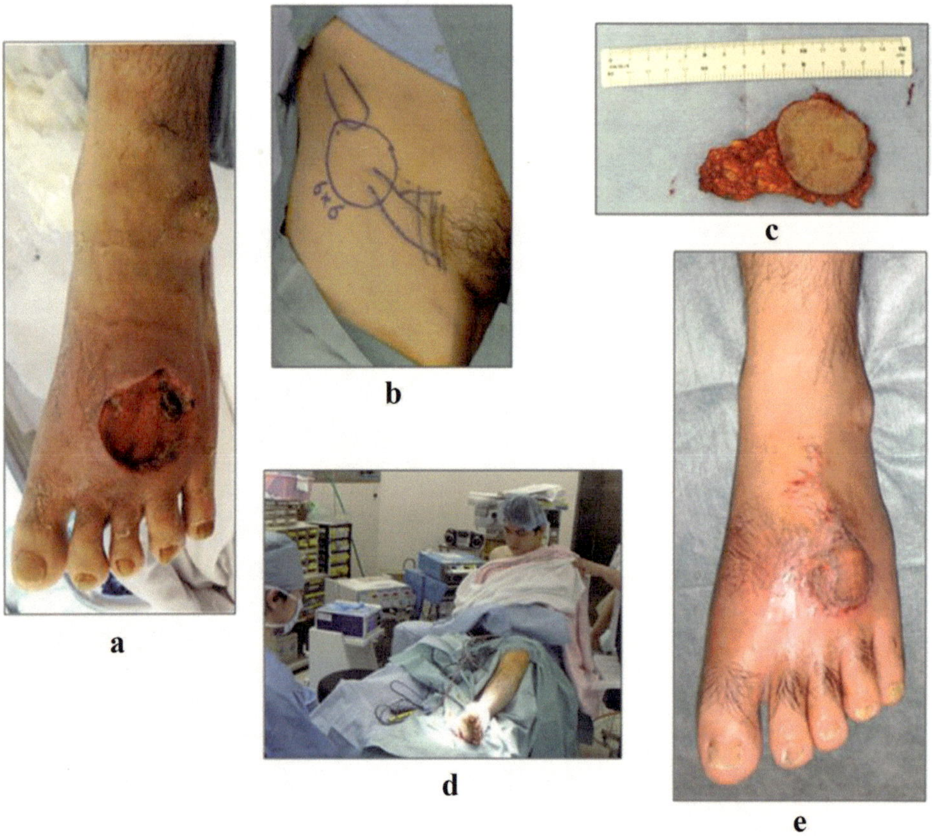

Figure 15.
(a) Case 4. A view of a diabetic foot ulcer of the step. (b) Intraoperative view showing the design of a free superficial circumflex iliac perforator flap. (c) Intraoperative view showing the design of a free SCIP flap. (d) Intraoperative view showing that an SCIP flap transfer is less invasive, so the patient was awake and talking with the surgeon. (e) A view of the reconstructed foot 2 months after surgery revealed favorable wound coverage.

be found near the wound [43]. Identifying an acceptable recipient vessel around the contaminated area is not always easy. Chronic inflammation in recipient vessels caused by infection and fibrosis may be one of the factors leading to thrombosis of the anastomosed vessel [44]. So, it is important to select a flap with a long pedicle, as the suitable recipient vessel may be distant from the wound. The *anterolateral thigh* (ATL) flap is often chosen because it is supplied by the descending branch of the lateral femoral circumflex artery, which has an external diameter of more than 2 mm at the proximal end with a pedicle of more than 8 cm in length [45, 46]. This flap is also a perforator flap, so that a larger cutaneous or fasciocutaneous flap can be harvested from the thigh while avoiding the sacrificing of underlying muscle and large vessels [47, 48].

Case presentation

Case 5. A 66-year-old man developed a diabetic foot ulcer with osteomyelitis of the left fourth and fifth toes (**Figure 16a**). He had already undergone right below

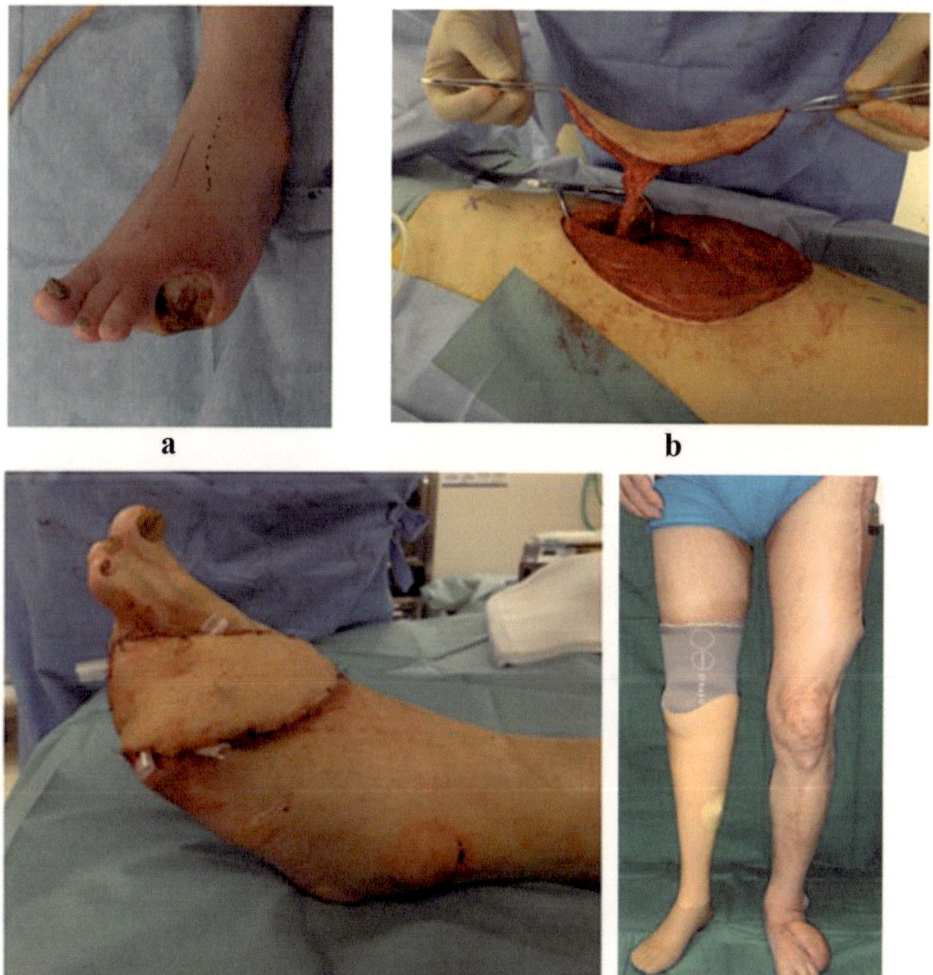

Figure 16.
(a) Case 5. A view of a diabetic foot ulcer. The fourth and fifth toes were amputated due to osteomyelitis. (b) Intraoperative view showing the elevation of an anterolateral thigh (ALT) flap. (c) Intraoperative view showing resurfacing of the bone-exposing wound with an ALT flap. (d) A view of the reconstructed foot 2 months after surgery revealed that favorable resurfacing had been achieved and he could walk without a cane.

the knee amputation due to diabetic gangrene. Thus, he desired to preserve his left leg to walk. Following debridement, he underwent resurfacing surgery using a free ALT flap (**Figure 16b** and **c**). Two months after the surgery, good resurfacing had been achieved, and he could walk with an artificial right leg (**Figure 16d**).

5. Conclusion

I conclude that the risk factors of leg amputation due to a diabetic foot are complications of severe infection and PAD, so diabetic ulcer management should include the immediate removal of necrotic tissue and control of infection. The only way to prevent major amputation of a diabetic ischemic foot is angioplasty of the occluded lower extremity arteries, and reconstruction of the amputation stump using free flap transfers to preserve the foot length is a good option for preserving the walking function.

Author details

Masaki Fujioka
Department of Plastic and Reconstructive Surgery, National Hospital Organization Nagasaki Medical Center, Ohmura City, Japan

*Address all correspondence to: inazumahayato7@gmail.com

References

[1] Vamos EP, Bottle A, Majeed A, Millett C. Trends in lower extremity amputations in people with and without diabetes in England, 1996-2005. Diabetes Research and Clinical Practice. 2010;**87**:275-282

[2] Lombardo FL, Maggini M, De Bellis A, Seghieri G, Anichini R. Lower extremity amputations in persons with and without diabetes in Italy: 2001-2010. PLoS One. 2014;**9**:e86405. Herder C, editor

[3] Lopez-de-Andres A, Jiménez-García R, Aragón-Sánchez J, Jiménez-Trujillo I, Hernández-Barrera V, Méndez-Bailón M, et al. National trends in incidence and outcomes in lower extremity amputations in people with and without diabetes in Spain, 2001-2012. Diabetes Research and Clinical Practice. 2015;**108**:499-507

[4] Watson MJ, Kundu N, Coppa C, Djohan R, Hashimoto K, Eghtesad B, et al. Role of tissue expanders in patients with loss of abdominal domain awaiting intestinal transplantation. Transplant International. 2013;**26**(12):1184-1190

[5] Fard B, Dijkstra PU, Stewart RE, Geertzen JHB. Incidence rates of dysvascular lower extremity amputation changes in Northern Netherlands: A comparison of three cohorts of 1991-1992, 2003-2004 and 2012-2013. PLoS One. 2018;**13**(9):e0204623

[6] Almaraz MC, González-Romero S, Bravo M, Caballero FF, Palomo MJ, Vallejo R, et al. Incidence of lower limb amputations in individuals with and without diabetes mellitus in Andalusia (Spain) from 1998 to 2006. Diabetes Research and Clinical Practice. 2012;**95**:399-405

[7] Qaseem A, Vijan S, Snow V, Cross JT, Weiss KB, Owens DK, et al. Glycemic control and type 2 diabetes mellitus: The optimal hemoglobin A1c targets. A guidance statement from the American College of Physicians. Annals of Internal Medicine. 2007;**147**:417-422

[8] van Houtum WH, Rauwerda JA, Ruwaard D, Schaper NC, Bakker K. Reduction in diabetes-related lower-extremity amputations in the Netherlands: 1991-2000. Diabetes Care. 2004;**27**:1042-1046

[9] Dabkana TM, Nyaku FT, Bwala ST. Current indications for extremity amputations in Maiduguri, North-East Nigeria: A 6-year retrospective review. Annals of African Medicine. 2018;**17**(1):22-25

[10] Yaghi K, Yaghi Y, McDonald AA, Yadegarfar G, Cecil E, Seidl J, et al. Diabetes or war? Incidence of and indications for limb amputation in Lebanon, 2007. Eastern Mediterranean Health Journal. 2012;**18**(12):1178-1186

[11] Sargen MR, Hoffstad O, Margolis DJ. Geographic variation in Medicare spending and mortality for diabetic patients with foot ulcers and amputations. Journal of Diabetes and its Complications. 2013;**27**(2):128-133

[12] Cook KD. Perioperative management of pedal amputations. Clinics in Podiatric Medicine and Surgery. 2005;**22**(3):329-341

[13] Zickler RW, Padberg FT Jr, Lal BK, Pappas PJ. When is a more proximal amputation needed? Clinics in Podiatric Medicine and Surgery. 2005;**22**(3):429-446

[14] Ammendola M, Sacco R, Butrico L, Sammarco G, de Franciscis S, Serra R. The care of transmetatarsal amputation in diabetic foot gangrene. International Wound Journal. 2017;**14**(1):9-15

[15] Pedersen NW, Pedersen D. Nutrition as a prognostic indicator in amputations. Acta Orthopaedica Scandinavica. 1992;**63**(6):675-678

[16] Ploeg AJ, Lardenoye JW, Vrancken Peeters MP, Breslau PJ. Contemporary series of morbidity and mortality after lower limb amputation. European Journal of Vascular and Endovascular Surgery. 2005;**29**(6):633-637

[17] Kay SP, Moreland JR, Schmitter E. Nutritional status and wound healing in lower extremity amputations. Clinical Orthopaedics and Related Research. 1987;**217**:253-256

[18] Luo H, Yang H, Huang B, Yuan D, Zhu J, Zhao J. Geriatric nutritional risk index (GNRI) independently predicts amputation inchronic criticallimb ischemia (CLI). PLoS One. 2016;**11**(3):e0152111

[19] Kawamura A, Horie T, Tsuda I, et al. Clinical study of therapeutic angiogenesis by autologous peripheral blood stem cell (PBSC) transplantation in 92 patients with critically ischemic limbs. Journal of Artificial Organs. 2006;**9**:226-233

[20] Iseki K. Pharmacological control of secondary hyperparathyroidism in chronic hemodialysis patients: Cinacalcet is coming to Japan. Expert Opinion on Pharmacotherapy. 2008;**9**:601-610

[21] Kaminski MR, Raspovic A, McMahon LP, Lambert KA, Erbas B, Mount PF, et al. Factors associated with foot ulceration and amputation in adults on dialysis: A cross-sectional observational study. BMC Nephrology. 2017;**18**(1):293

[22] Bencini PL, Montagnino G, Citterio A, Graziani G, Crosti C, Ponticelli C. Cutaneous abnormalities in uremic patients. Nephron. 1985;**40**:3163-3121

[23] Pico MR, Lugo-Somolinos A. Cutaneous alterations in patients with chronic renal failure. International Journal of Dermatology. 1992;**31**:860-863

[24] Wukich DK, Ahn J, Raspovic KM, Gottschalk FA, La Fontaine J, Lavery LA.Comparison of transtibial amputations in diabetic patients with and without end-stage renal disease. Foot & Ankle International. 2017;**38**(4):388-396

[25] Vas PRJ, Edmonds M, Kavarthapu V, Rashid H, Ahluwalia R, Pankhurst C, et al. The diabetic foot attack: "Tis too late to retreat!". The International Journal of Lower Extremity Wounds. 2018;**17**(1):7-13

[26] Fujioka M. More than half of patients receiving hemodialysis with leg ulcer require amputation. In: Suzuki H, editor. Hemodialysis. Rijeka: InTech; 2013. pp. P231-P240

[27] Garimella PS, Wang W, Lin SF, Hymes J, Lacson E Jr. Incident diabetic foot ulcers and mortality in hemodialysis patients. Hemodialysis International. 2017;**21**(1):145-147

[28] Marn Pernat A, Peršič V, Usvyat L, Saunders L, Rogus J, Maddux FW, et al. Implementation of routine foot check in patients with diabetes on hemodialysis: Associations with outcomes. BMJ Open Diabetes Research & Care. 2016;**4**(1):e000158

[29] Mustățea P, Bugă C, Doran H, Mihalache O, Bobîrcă FT, Georgescu DE, et al. Soft tissue infections in diabetic patients. Chirurgia (Bucharest). 2018;**113**(5):651-667

[30] Lavery LA, Davis KE, Berriman SJ, Braun L, Nichols A, Kim PJ, et al. WHS guidelines update: Diabetic foot ulcer treatment guidelines. Wound Repair and Regeneration. 2016;**24**(1):112-126

[31] Perren S, Gatt A, Papanas N, Formosa C. Hyperbaric oxygen therapy in ischaemic foot ulcers in type 2 diabetes: A clinical trial. Open Cardiovascular Medicine Journal. 2018;**12**:80-85

[32] Erdoğan A, Düzgün AP, Erdoğan K, Özkan MB, Coşkun F. Efficacy of hyperbaric oxygen therapy in diabetic foot ulcers based on Wagner classification. The Journal of Foot and Ankle Surgery. 2018;**57**(6):1115-1119

[33] Tchero H, Kangambega P, Noubou L, Becsangele B, Fluieraru S, Teot L. Antibiotic therapy of diabetic foot infections: A systematic review of randomized controlled trials. Wound Repair and Regeneration. Sep 2018;**26**(5):381-391

[34] Hinchliffe RJ, Brownrigg JR, Andros G, Apelqvist J, Boyko EJ, Fitridge R, et al. International Working Group on the Diabetic Foot. Effectiveness of revascularization of the ulcerated foot in patients with diabetes and peripheral artery disease: A systematic review. Diabetes/Metabolism Research and Reviews. 2016;**32**(Suppl 1):136-144

[35] Forsythe RO, Brownrigg J, Hinchliffe RJ. Peripheral arterial disease and revascularization of the diabetic foot. Diabetes, Obesity & Metabolism. 2015;**17**(5):435-444

[36] Vouillarmet J, Bourron O, Gaudric J, Lermusiaux P, Millon A, Hartemann A. Lower-extremity arterial revascularization: Is there any evidence for diabetic foot ulcer-healing? Diabetes & Metabolism. 2016;**42**(1):4-15

[37] Hahn HM, Jeong KS, Park MC, Park DH, Lee IJ. Free-flap transfer for coverage of transmetatarsal amputation stump to preserve residual foot length. The International Journal of Lower Extremity Wounds. 2017;**16**(1):60-65

[38] Baumfeld D, Baumfeld T, Macedo B, Zambelli R, Lopes F, Nery C. Factors related to amputation level and wound healing in diabetic patients. Acta Ortopedica Brasileira. 2018;**26**(5):342-345

[39] El-Sabbagh AH. Skin perforator flaps: An algorithm for leg reconstruction. Journal of Reconstructive Microsurgery. 2011;**27**:511-523

[40] Parrett BM, Matros E, Pribaz JJ, et al. Lower extremity trauma: Trends in the management of soft-tissue reconstruction of open tibia-fibula fractures. Plastic and Reconstructive Surgery. 2006;**117**:1315-1322

[41] Schaverien M, Saint-Cyr M. Perforators of the lower leg: Analysis of perforator locations and clinical application for pedicled perforator flaps. Plastic and Reconstructive Surgery. 2008;**122**:161-170

[42] Taylor GI, Pan WR. Angiosomes of the leg: Anatomic study and clinical implications. Plastic and Reconstructive Surgery. 1998;**102**:599-616

[43] Suh YC, Hong JP, Suh HP. Elevation technique for medial branch based superficial circumflex iliac artery perforator flap. Handchirurgie, Mikrochirurgie, Plastische Chirurgie. 2018;**50**(4):256-258

[44] Rudolph R, Arganese T, Woodward M. The ultrastructure and etiology of chronic radiotherapy damage in human skin. Annals of Plastic Surgery. 1982;**9**(4):282-292

[45] Wong CH, Wei FC. Anterolateral thigh flap. Head & Neck. 2010;**32**(4):529-540

[46] Wei FC, Jain V, Celik N, Chen HC, Chuang DC, Lin CH. Have we found an ideal soft-tissue flap? An experience with 672 anterolateral thigh flaps. Plastic and Reconstructive Surgery. 2002;**109**:2219-2226

[47] Fujioka M. Application of Free Flow-through Anterolateral Thigh Flap for the Reconstruction of an Extremity Soft Tissue Defect Requiring Vascularization. Flap Surgery. Rijeka: InTech; 2018. pp. 51-76. Chapter 4

[48] Gokhan M, Ulusal AE, Atik A, Sargin S, Ulusal B, Sukru Sahin M. Descending branch of the lateral circumflex femoral artery as a recipient vessel for vascularized fibular grafts: Clinical case series. Microsurgery. 2014;**34**(8):633-637

Chapter 3

Multidisciplinary Management of Severe Extremity Injuries

Mitsuru Nemoto

Abstract

Management of severe extremity injuries begins with controlling bleeding and stabilizing hemodynamics. There is no agreement regarding the selection of amputation or limb salvage for severe extremity injuries. The injury severity scoring system should be carefully and judiciously used. The important factor for the management of open fractures is how early the injured area of soft tissues is covered. Inappropriate management would increase complications and prolong the treatment period. Multidisciplinary management by specialists, in the emergency department, orthopedics, plastic surgery, vascular surgery, and rehabilitation, insisting on employing their own individual abilities as much as possible, would not only help to salvage limbs in severe extremity injuries but also provide highly satisfactory functional and aesthetic outcomes for patients.

Keywords: severe extremity injury, management, reconstruction, salvage, amputation

1. Introduction

The goal of treatment for severe extremity injuries is limb salvage; however, complicated life-threatening injuries and mangled extremities may lead to indication of amputation. To achieve an optimal outcome in patients with severe extremity injuries requires multidisciplinary management that begins with resuscitation and evaluation of life-threatening injuries, following initial surgical management, definitive treatment, and postoperative care. Initial surgical management includes control of bleeding sites by vascular ligation and/or shunting, debridement of devitalized soft tissues and foreign materials, and stabilization of the fracture by external fixation. Definitive treatment includes internal fixation of long bones, vessel reconstruction with anastomosis and/or grafts, nerve repair, and soft tissue coverage within the appropriate time frame. This chapter describes the multidisciplinary management of severe extremity injuries based on the morphological and functional characteristics of upper and lower extremities.

2. Initial assessment and management

Initial assessment begins with the primary survey, in which the patients' life-threatening injuries are evaluated based on the Advanced Trauma Life Support (ATLS) manual [1]. Establishment of an airway to avoid asphyxiation, maintenance and management of breathing, and circulation management by hemostatic procedure, and possibly transfusion, should be performed. Persistent bleeding should be detected early. Elastic or compression bandage or tourniquet is used when the bleeding cannot be stopped directly. Examination for bleeding sites in other regions than the extremities should be made. After the patient has been made hemodynamically stable, the next step is the secondary survey in which injuries are systematically surveyed to determine whether or not they require immediate medical treatment.

3. Extremity evaluation

The most important thing in the initial examination of extremity injuries is to evaluate whether or not the injuries are life-threatening and/or if they could cause dysfunctions. Meanwhile, if there are life-threatening complications, the initial diagnoses of minor injuries such as fractures with slight deformity or dislocation and/or ligament injuries are difficult and often likely to be missed. To preserve function of the extremities, the evaluation should be performed with careful attention to the maintenance of blood flow in the extremities, prevention of infection, proper treatment of surrounding skin and soft tissue injuries, and the prevention of secondary injuries. Tests of sensibility, motor function of and pulse in the bilateral extremities are periodically performed and recorded.

3.1 Peripheral nerve assessment

Systematic neurological assessment is essential. Sites exhibiting paresthesia, their distribution, and the ability of locomotor activity of muscles innervated by the peripheral nervous system should be examined. Muscle strength is evaluated by manual muscle testing. Definitive diagnosis can be made by examining the lesions in the operating room and confirming the presence or absence of any nerve injuries. However, in the case of blunt nerve injuries, often making a diagnosis is not easy, even when the lesion is open. In such cases, electrical nerve stimulation and observation of funiculus with an operating microscope would help in making a diagnosis. Especially in patients with multiple injuries, evaluation of nervous function is often initially difficult. Repetitive reevaluations should be made concurrently with the other surveys after the patient's condition has been stabilized.

3.2 Vascular assessment

Extremity vascular injuries are classified into two groups depending on the type of causes: penetrating injuries made by knives and such, and blunt injuries due to fractures, dislocations, etc. Delay of diagnosis and treatment for extremity major arterial injuries influences the functional prognosis. Especially, blunt injuries of lower limb arteries often require fasciotomy and/or amputation and are associated with higher mortality [2]. Therefore, to avoid sequelae (e.g., residual disability) associated with extremity arterial injuries, early and accurate diagnosis is indispensable.

When right and left difference in peripheral artery pulsation or skin color, continuous bleeding, and/or the sign of an expanding hematoma are observed after an injury, extremity arterial injury is suspected. However, because there are some cases that in spite of the extremity major artery injury, apparent ischemic signs cannot be initially seen due to the presence of a collateral circulation, extra careful attention is required. For the diagnosis of extremity arterial injuries, examinations by Doppler-derived arterial pressure measurement [3, 4] and helical CT angiography [5, 6] are adopted.

Diagnosis of the presence or absence of arterial injuries should not be made easily only by the evaluation of the capillary return sign and/or the Doppler-derived arterial pressure measurement. Suspected patients should undergo early angiography for a definitive diagnosis of the presence or absence of arterial injuries. However, revascularization should not be delayed due to putting a high priority on angiography. If ischemia due to arterial injury is suspected, early revascularization is necessary to save limbs, so it is also necessary to take surgery with information of the minimum contrast CT.

3.3 Soft tissue and bone assessment

When open injuries are found on the skin and soft tissues, diagnosis is easy from local findings. However, closed injuries of the skin and soft tissues are likely to be missed. When pulsation, mobility, dysesthesia, tire mark, and/or cutaneous abrasions are found on the skin, closed injuries are suspected. Open wounds should not be washed out before coming to the hospital or before debridement at the emergency department, because bacterial culture swabs are taken from the open wound. Then antibiotics are rapidly administered by infusion for the prevention of infection and a tetanus inoculation should be given. The administration of antibiotics from the prehospital period might help to lower the risk of infection at the site of a severe open fracture [7]. The confirmation procedure to determine whether or not the open wound, even if small, is in the communicating area of the fracture is performed under proper anesthesia in an operating room.

In the treatment of amputated extremities, tissues are wrapped with saline-soaked gauze, put into a plastic bag, and stored in ice water at 4°C.

3.4 Injury severity score

When we have to decide amputation or limb salvage depending on the degree of injury, the severity of extremity injury is evaluated based on the extremity assessment. Severity evaluation systems are the Gustilo-Anderson classification (**Table 1**) [8, 9], the Mangled Extremity Syndrome Index [10], the Predictive Salvage Index System [11], the Mangled Extremity Severe Score (MESS) (**Table 2**) [12], the Limb Salvage Index [13], and NISSSA (Nerve Injury, Ischemia, Soft Tissue Injury, Skeletal Injury, Shock, and Age of the patient) Score [14]. Among them, the Gustilo-Anderson classification and MESS are well-known severity evaluation systems. Although the Gustilo-Anderson classification is essentially designed to apply to

Gustilo-Anderson Classification
Type I
Open fracture is transverse or short oblique fracture with minimal comminution
Wound is less than 1 cm with minimal soft tissue injury
Type II
Open fracture is simple transverse or short oblique fracture with minimal comminution
Wound is greater than 1 cm with moderate soft tissue injury
Type IIIA
Adequate soft tissue coverage of a fractured bone despite extensive soft tissue laceration or flaps, or high-energy trauma irrespective of wound size
Type IIIB
Extensive soft tissue injury loss with periosteal stripping and bone exposure
Usually associated with massive contamination
Wound requires local or free flap coverage
Type IIIC
Open fracture associated with arterial injury requiring repair, regardless of degree of soft tissue injury

Table 1.
Gustilo-Anderson classification.

	Points
Skeletal / soft-tissue injury	
Low energy (stab; simple fracture; civilian gunshot wound)	1
Medium energy (open or multiple fractures, dislocation)	2
High energy (close-range gunshot or military gunshot wound, crush injury)	3
Very high energy (above + gross contamination, soft tissue avulsion)	4
Limb ischemia	
Pulse reduced or absent but perfusion normal, less than 6 hours	1
Pulse reduced or absent but perfusion normal, more than 6 hours	2
Pulseless; paresthesias, diminished capillary refill for less than 6 hours	2
Pulseless; paresthesias, diminished capillary refill for more than 6 hours	4
Cool, paralyzed, insensate, numb extremity for less than 6 hours	3
Cool, paralyzed, insensate, numb extremity for more than 6 hours	6
Shock	
Systolic BP always > 90 mm Hg	0
Hypotensive transiently	1
Persistent hypotension	2
Age (years)	
< 30	0
30-50	1
> 50	2

Table 2.
Mangled Extremity Severity Score (MESS).

intraoperative findings, it is actually often used from the initial evaluation. This classification method provides indices for the infection rate and the bone union period following the treatment of open fractures. MESS is composed of injury mechanism, severity and duration of limb ischemia, severity of shock, and patient's age. When the score is ≥7, amputation is likely to be selected [15–18].

4. Surgical management

Surgical management for extremity injuries is performed under the condition of stable hemodynamics with controlled bleeding. The management procedures include damage control surgery, fracture management, revascularization, extremity fasciotomy, nerve repair, and soft tissue debridement and coverage. When the bleeding cannot be controlled in an unrepairable extremity injury, limb amputation is selected.

4.1 Damage control surgery

If bleeding from the extremities continues, it is stopped by compression. If the compression does not work, bleeding is controlled using tourniquet and damaged blood vessels are treated by ligation or vascular repair. Patients should undergo revascularization within 6 hours, and if the ischemic time is prolonged, vascular shunt should be constructed. If the arteries and veins are both damaged, shunting is required for each artery and vein. However, if it is impossible, veins are occluded by ligation.

4.2 Fracture management

When the open fracture of extremities is severe, debridement and skeletal stabilization are performed in the operating room after the evaluation and stabilization of concomitant injuries that could be life-threatening. For the initial skeletal stabilization, external fixation is useful.

4.2.1 Debridement and stabilization

At the initial surgery, thorough debridement of mangled tissues and foreign bodies is performed. Low-pressure irrigation is used for the lavage. A delay in the debridement is likely to lead to high rate of infection and/or amputation [19–21]. The grade of the Gustilo-Anderson classification is evaluated by the assessment of conditions of conserved soft tissues and fractures. It is difficult to accurately evaluate the grade of the soft tissue injuries and the presence or absence of infection at the initial surgery. In most cases, a second-look and/or third-look debridement is required. External fixation is often selected as the initial skeletal stabilization for severe open fractures. When there are major vessel injuries, prompt skeletal stabilization and revascularization should be required. If it takes a long time for skeletal stabilization, a vascular shunt should be made to shorten the ischemic time. The defect of the surrounding soft tissues is reevaluated within 72 hours in the operating room, and additional debridement or definitive fracture fixation and soft tissue coverage are performed.

4.2.2 Definitive fracture fixation

Definitive fracture fixation is performed when the patient's condition, even with concomitant injuries, is stable. It is ideal that for the treatment of open fractures, external fixation has been changed to internal fixation, and soft tissue defects are promptly covered. For relatively low-grade open fractures of long bones, fixation with intramedullary nailing is considered preferable. However, because there is little difference in the outcomes between reamed and unreamed medullary nailing for long bone open fractures, the benefit of these procedures remains controversial [22–24]. External fixation of fractures offers a safe and effective management option for children (**Figure 1**) [25].

4.3 Revascularization

Factors influencing the functional prognosis after the main extremity artery injuries are proper treatment of the fracture and soft tissue injuries, including the nervous system, and the length of ischemic time. Because irreversible degeneration of muscle tissues is caused by ischemia of 6 hours or longer, the period between injury and revascularization should be as short as possible. The revascularization procedure includes vascular repair, vein grafting, inserting bypasses, stents, and/or shunts, which should be performed by surgeons with extensive experience in treating such injuries. When there are multiple levels of vessel injuries, revascularization should be started caudally from the most proximal vessel to the injury. If revascularization is likely to take up to 4 hours or longer, a temporary shunt should be constructed. In severe extremity injuries, revascularization after constructing a temporary shunt will decrease the amputation rates (**Figure 2**) [26]. When there is a defect of the vessels or the tension in the anastomotic site is strong, revascularization is performed after vein grafting (**Figure 3**). When there is a problem with venous return due to the injuries, revascularization of veins is performed.

4.4 Extremity fasciotomy

The fracture and bruising cause the muscles to swell, and the inner pressure of fascial compartments to rise. The compartment syndrome is the state that muscles are swollen further with lowered perfusion pressure, and the nervous system and muscles become ischemic. Diagnosis is determined from the present medical history

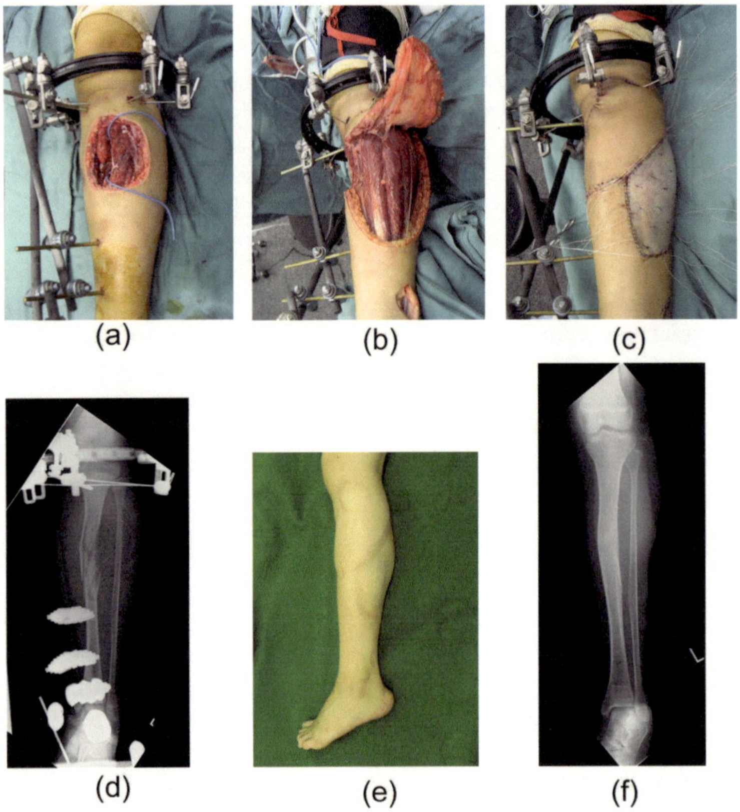

Figure 1.
(a) Open fracture of the left lower extremity was accompanied by a moderate soft tissue defect on the anterior lower extremity. (b) The fasciocutaneous flap was elevated from the lateral side. (c) Moderate soft tissue defect was covered by a fasciocutaneous flap, and skin grafting was applied to the donor site. (d) Intraoperative X-ray. (e) Postoperative view 84 months after surgery. (f) An X-ray of the leg 84 months after surgery, showing good bone union.

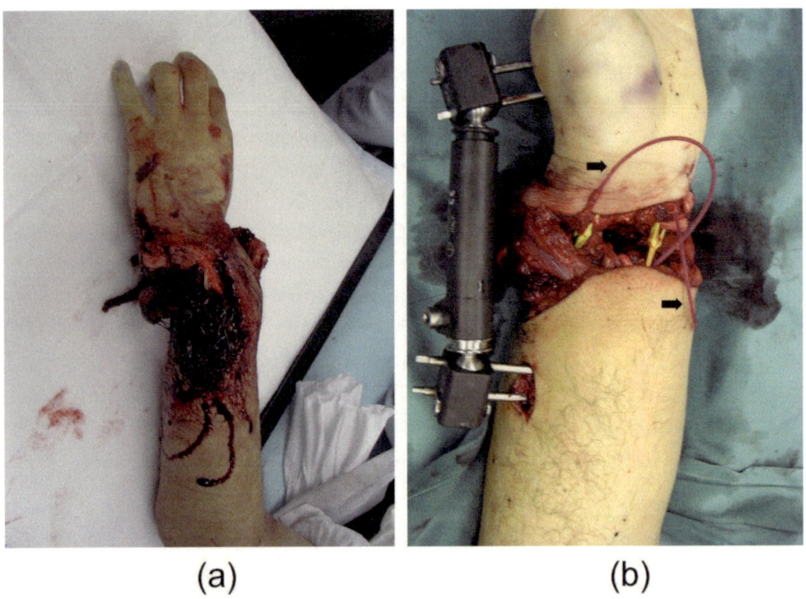

Figure 2.
(a) Crush injury of the left forearm was accompanied by injuries to the radial and ulnar arteries. (b) Temporary vascular shunts (arrowheads) were placed into the radial and ulnar arteries before definitive vascular repair.

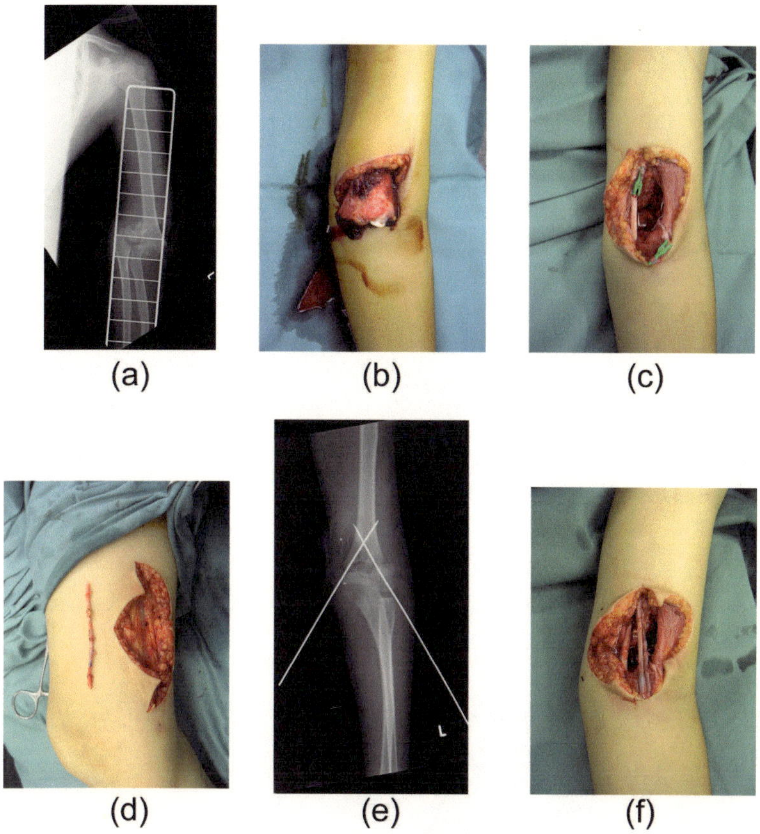

Figure 3.
(a) Preoperative X-ray. (b, c) The supracondylar fracture is accompanied by brachial vessel injuries. (d) The saphenous vein was harvested from the right thigh. (e) X-ray findings after Kirchner wire fixation, intraoperatively. (f) The saphenous vein was cut in half, and then the two veins were interposed in way of grafting to repair the defects in the brachial artery and vein.

and findings in physical examinations. Signs and symptoms are swelling in the overall area of the injury site, severe pain that cannot be alleviated by analgesics, increase of pain in the stretch test, and dysesthesia in the compartment region. Even though the compartment syndrome develops, peripheral arterial pulsation is usually palpable. During 48 hours after the injury, clinical signs and symptoms are periodically checked. Because clinical signs and symptoms cannot be checked if the patients have impaired consciousness or are under the effect of sedatives, inner pressure of the compartment is measured if the compartment syndrome is suspected. When the compartment inner pressure is ≥35–40 mmHg, a fasciotomy is performed (**Figure 4**). The open wound after a fasciotomy is treated by delayed primary closure and/or skin graft.

4.5 Nerve repair

Nerve injury that occurs concomitantly with fractures and/or dislocations is treated by repositioning and simple fixation. It is important that nerve repair is carefully performed using an operating microscope or surgical loupes. Factors other than surgery, such as the patient's age, nerve injury at higher level, and the degree of injury, influence the recovery of nerve damage. In cases with life-threatening concomitant injuries and/or those with severe extremity injuries, nerve repair can be performed later, within 2 weeks, with good prognoses. If the torn nerve fiber can be identified, marking with a nylon suture at the end of the nerve fiber or fibers is

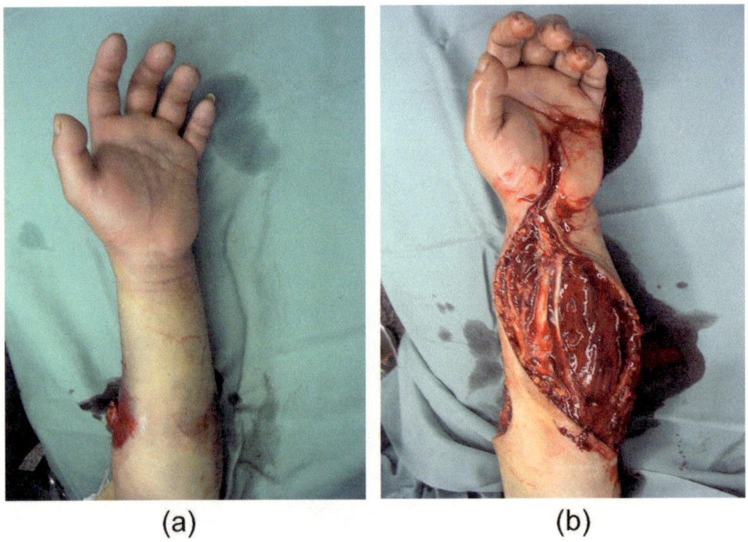

Figure 4.
(a) The left forearm was wringed by a industrial press machine, and the injury progressed to the compartment syndrome. (b) Fasciotomy was performed to alleviate the compartment pressure.

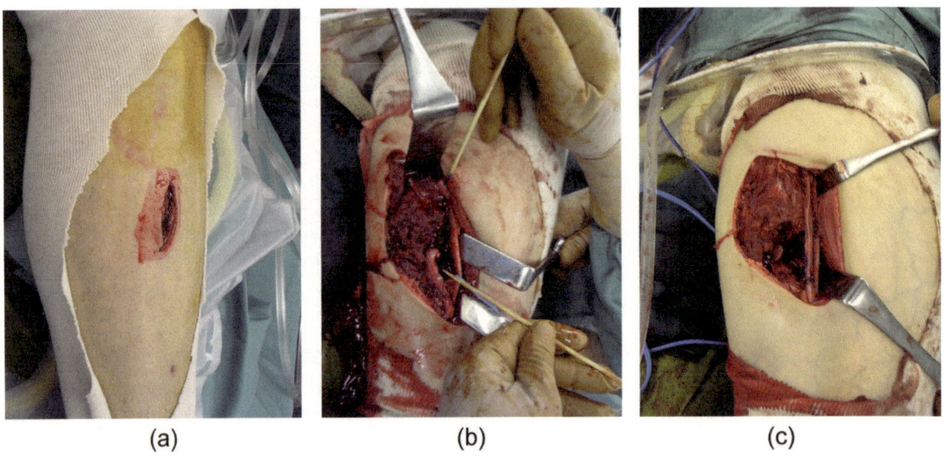

Figure 5.
(a) A penetrating wound was located in the middle of the right thigh. (b) The tibial nerve was ablated and crushed. (c) The sural nerve was divided in thirds and used as a cable graft to repair the severed tibial nerve.

recommended for later surgical repair. To treat a complete tear of nerve fibers, the nerve fibers are sutured together after the cut ends are reinnervated. When there is a high tension at the suture site or suturing is difficult or impossible because of nerve gaps, autologous nerve grafting [27] (**Figure 5**) or reconstruction with artificial nerve conduit [28] is incorporated into the treatment.

4.6 Soft tissue debridement and definitive coverage

In open fractures, the degree of soft tissue injury is associated with prognosis [29]. Soft tissue wounds in severe extremity injuries have a high risk of infection and treatment should be begun immediately. There have been a few reports on immediate wound closure and primary wound closure [30–32]. However, because it is difficult to accurately evaluate the degree of soft tissue damage and the presence or absence of

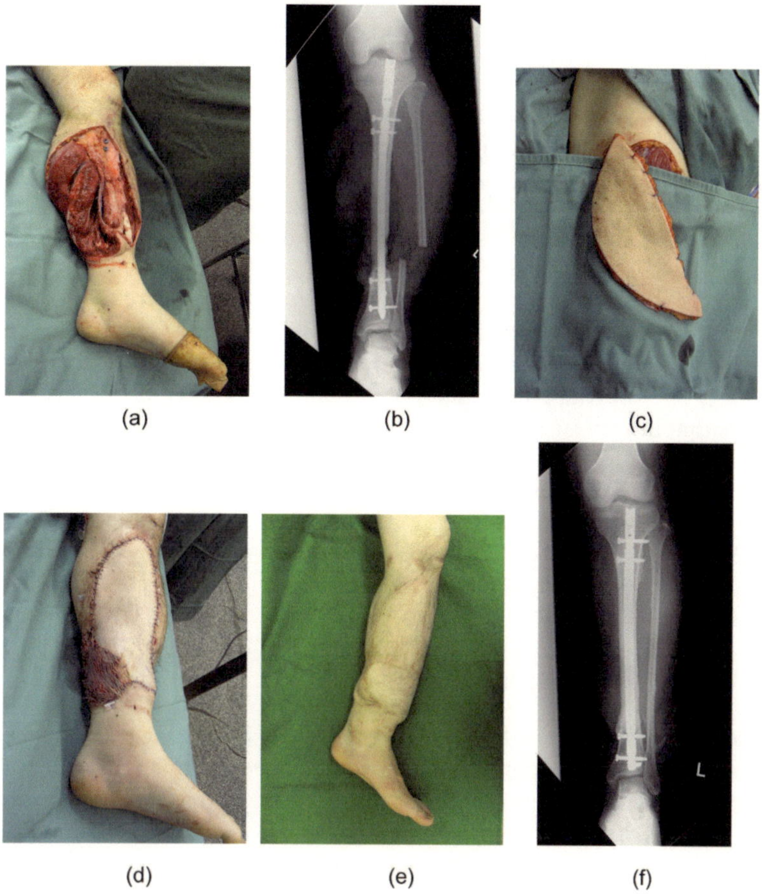

Figure 6.
(a) An open fracture located in the distal third of the left lower extremity, accompanied by massive soft tissue defect. (b) Intraoperative X-ray after intramedullary nailing fixation. (c) The anterolateral thigh fasciocutaneous flap was harvested from the right thigh. (d) The anterolateral thigh fasciocutaneous flap was applied to the soft tissue defect. Six months after internal fixation, autogenous bone grafting and transposition of the fasciocutaneous flap was performed on the tibia defect. (e) Postoperative view 12 months after bone grafting. (f) X-ray at 12-month follow-up showing adequate bone union.

infection in severe extremity injuries, the number of cases in which immediate wound closure and primary wound closure are possible is limited. In most cases with severe extremity injuries, second-look and/or third-look debridement are required. Open wounds had been recommended to be treated with moist dressings after debridement. Recently, although NPWT (negative pressure wound therapy) is used for open fracture wounds during the period after the debridement until coverage [33], there has been no evidence that it is more useful than conventional moist dressing [34, 35].

Because the infection rate becomes higher with the passage of days after the injury of an open fracture, the open wound should be closed early if the patient's general condition is stable and there is no local infection [36, 37]. For the coverage of the defect of soft tissues after the bone fixation, a flap is recommended [36–41]. Even if wound coverage cannot be performed at the initial debridement, good functional prognosis can be expected when soft tissue coverage is performed within 72 hours after an injury [36, 38, 40]. For an extensive soft tissue defect, a free flap transfer is useful (**Figure 6**). A free flap transfer enables reconstruction of a soft tissue defect by an end to side or a flow-through type vascular anastomosis without sacrificing major vessels, even if the recipient vessels that can be anastomosed are limited [42].

5. Complications

Complications associated with severe extremity injuries include infection and/or necrosis, pseudoarthrosis, osteomyelitis, venous thromboembolism, and rhabdomyolysis. If these complications occur, additional treatment is required and the treatment period would be prolonged.

5.1 Wound complications

Wound complications are caused by insufficient debridement and/or infection. The infection rate becomes higher with a higher grade of the Gustilo-Anderson classification. To prevent infection in severe extremity injuries, it is important to perform early and thorough debridement of necrotic tissues and construct coverage with tissues that have abundant blood flow.

5.2 Venous thromboembolism

Deep vein thrombosis (DVT) and pulmonary embolism (PE) occur in 2–58% of trauma patients [43–45]. Because severe extremity injuries have a high risk of DVT and PE, mechanical and pharmacologic prophylaxes are necessary [46].

5.3 Rhabdomyolysis and myoglobinuria

Rhabdomyolysis and myoglobinuria are observed in the crush syndrome, compartment syndrome, and reperfusion syndrome. Various substances released from necrotic striated muscle cells circulate throughout the body, causing hyperkalemia, metabolic acidosis, hypermyoglobinemia, and acute renal failure. Transfusion and correction of electrolytes are fundamental to preventing acute renal failure.

6. Amputation versus limb salvage

There is, as yet, no agreement on the selection criteria for amputation or limb salvage [47–49]. The injury severity scoring system is reported to be a good indictor in a few reports [50–53] but considered negatively in others [54–56]. Because the indications for amputation differ depending on the patient's age (whether an adult or a child), and occupation, the injury severity scoring system should be used carefully and judiciously [57–60]. Indications for amputation are as follows: (1) life-threatening

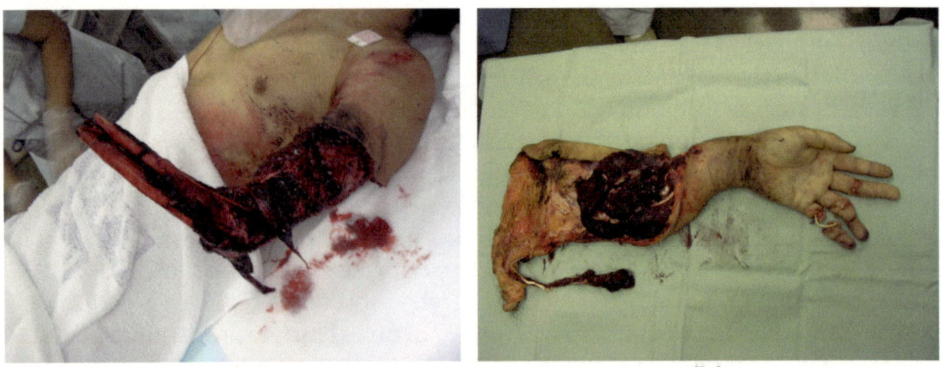

(a) (b)

Figure 7.
(a and b) The left upper extremity was avulsed by an industrial machine. This mangled limb was not salvageable.

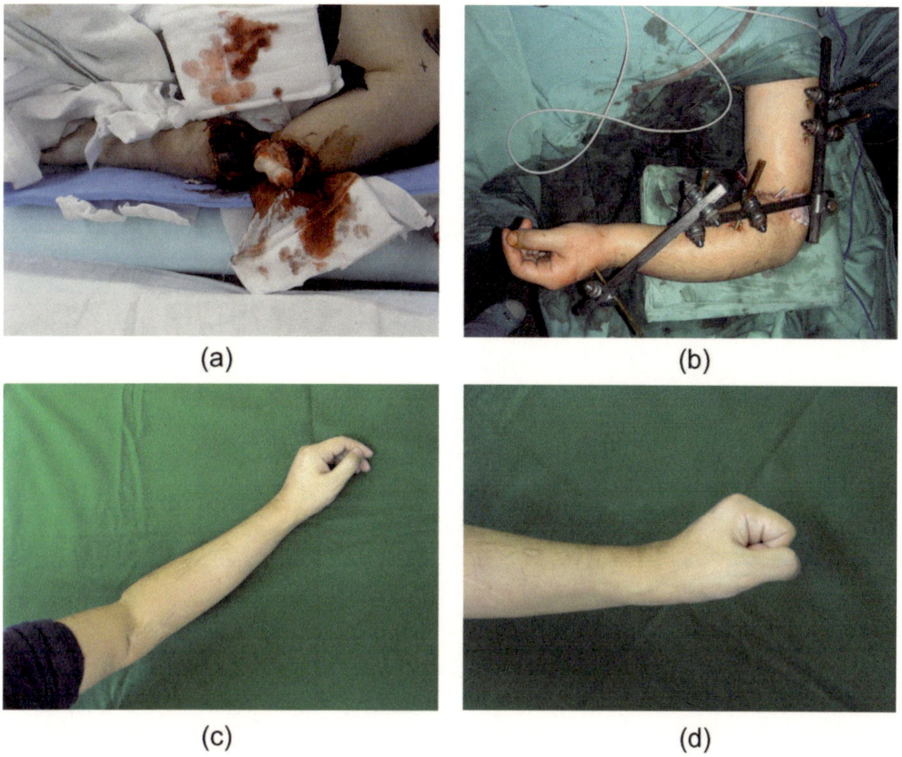

Figure 8.
(a) The left upper extremity was ablated at the elbow, the median and ulnar nerves were preserved; however, the radial nerve was avulsed in the middle third of the upper arm. (b) Immediate revascularization to the brachial vessels was performed followed by external fixation. (c and d) Postoperative view 12 months after reconstruction and a modified Riordan operation was performed on the radial nerve to cure the palsy.

bleeding cannot be controlled, (2) preserving open injuries to the extremity is likely to cause the patients' mortality, and (3) the injuries are so severe that a specialist judges the salvage of the extremity to be impossible (**Figure 7**). Ultimately, the decision regarding choosing limb salvage or amputation should be made in discussion with the patients themselves and their family members (**Figure 8**). Primary delayed amputation, if deemed necessary, should be performed within 72 hours after the injury.

7. Conclusions

For the treatment of severe extremity injuries, multidisciplinary management is required from the primary survey through rehabilitation. Unless severe extremity injuries are treated properly within the proper time frames, complications may occur, resulting in severe sequelae. Multidisciplinary management by specialists, in the emergency department, orthopedics, plastic surgery, vascular surgery, and rehabilitation, insisting on employing their own individual abilities as much as possible, would not only help to salvage limbs in severe extremity injuries but also provide highly satisfactory functional and aesthetic outcomes for patients.

Conflict of interest

The author declares that there is no conflict of interest regarding the publication of this chapter.

Author details

Mitsuru Nemoto
Department of Plastic and Aesthetic Surgery, Kitasato University School of Medicine, Japan

*Address all correspondence to: mnemoto@med.kitasato-u.ac.jp

References

[1] American College of Surgeons Committee on Trauma. Advanced Trauma Life Support (ATLS) Student Course Manual. 9th ed. Chicago: American College of Surgeons; 2012

[2] Tan TW, Joglar FL, Hamburg NM, et al. Limb outcome and mortality in lower and upper extremity arterial injury: A comparison using the National Trauma Data Bank. Vascular and Endovascular Surgery. 2011;**45**:592-597. DOI: 10.1177/1538574411415125

[3] Lynch K, Johansen K. Can Doppler pressure measurement replace "exclusion" arteriography in the diagnosis of occult extremity arterial trauma? Annals of Surgery. 1991;**214**:737-741

[4] Mills WJ, Barei DP, McNair P. The value of the ankle-brachial index for diagnosing arterial injury after knee dislocation: A prospective study. The Journal of Trauma. 2004;**56**:1261-1265

[5] Soto JA, Munera F, Cardoso N, et al. Diagnostic performance of helical CT angiography in trauma to large arteries of the extremities. Journal of Computer Assisted Tomography. 1999;**23**:188-196

[6] Busquets AR, Acosta JA, Colon E, et al. Helical computed tomographic angiography for the diagnosis of traumatic arterial injuries of the extremities. The Journal of Trauma. 2004;**56**:625-628

[7] Lack WD, Karunakar MA, Angerame MR, et al. Type III open tibia fractures: Immediate antibiotic prophylaxis minimizes infection. Journal of Orthopaedic Trauma. 2015;**29**:1-6. DOI: 10.1097/BOT.0000000000000262

[8] Gustilo RB, Anderson JT. Prevention of infection in the treatment of one thousand and twenty-five open fractures of long bones: Retrospective and prospective analyses. The Journal of Bone and Joint Surgery. 1976;**58**:453-458

[9] Gustilo RB, Mendoza RM, Williams DN. Problems in the management of type III (severe) open fractures: A new classification of type III open fractures. The Journal of Trauma. 1984;**24**:742-746

[10] Gregory RT, Gould RJ, Peclet M, et al. The mangled extremity syndrome (M.E.S.): A severity grading system for multisystem injury of the extremity. The Journal of Trauma. 1985;**25**:1147-1150

[11] Howe HR Jr, Poole GV Jr, Hansen KJ, et al. Salvage of lower extremities following combined orthopedic and vascular trauma. A predictive salvage index. The American Surgeon. 1987;**53**:205-208

[12] Johansen K, Daines M, Howey T, et al. Objective criteria accurately predict amputation following lower extremity trauma. The Journal of Trauma. 1990;**30**:568-573

[13] Russell WL, Sailors DM, Whittle TB, et al. Limb salvage versus traumatic amputation. A decision based on a seven-part predictive index. Annals of Surgery. 1991;**213**:473-480

[14] McNamara MG, Heckman JD, Corley FG. Severe open fractures of the lower extremity: A retrospective evaluation of the mangled extremity severity score (MESS). Journal of Orthopaedic Trauma. 1994;**8**:81-87

[15] Behdad S, Rafiei MH, Taheri H, et al. Evaluation of mangled extremity severity score (MESS) as a predictor of lower limb amputation in children with trauma. European Journal of Pediatric Surgery. 2012;**22**:465-469. DOI: 10.1055/s-0032-1322541

[16] Kumar MK, Badole C, Patond K. Salvage versus amputation: Utility of

mangled extremity severity score in severely injured lower limbs. Indian Journal of Orthopaedics. 2007;**41**: 183-187. DOI: 10.4103/0019-5413.33679

[17] Rush RM Jr, Kjorstad R, Starnes BW, et al. Application of the mangled extremity severity score in a combat setting. Military Medicine. 2007;**172**:777-781

[18] Robertson PA. Prediction of amputation after severe lower limb trauma. Journal of Bone and Joint Surgery. 1991;**73**:816-818

[19] Sears ED, Davis MM, Chung KC. Relationship between timing of emergency procedures and limb amputation in patients with open tibia fracture in the United States, 2003 to 2009. Plastic and Reconstructive Surgery. 2012;**130**:369-378. DOI: 10.1097/PRS.0b013e3182589e2d

[20] Hull PD, Johnson SC, Stephen DJ, et al. Delayed debridement of severe open fractures is associated with a higher rate of deep infection. The Bone & Joint Journal. 2014;**96**:379-384. DOI: 10.1302/0301-620x.96B3.32380

[21] Malhotra AK, Goldberg S, Graham J, et al. Open extremity fractures: Impact of delay in operative debridement and irrigation. Journal of Trauma and Acute Care Surgery. 2014;**76**:1201-1207. DOI: 10.1097/TA.0000000000000205

[22] Keating JF, O'Brien PJ, Blachut PA, et al. Locking intramedullary nailing with and without reaming for open fractures of the tibial shaft. A prospective, randomized study. The Journal of Bone and Joint Surgery. 1997;**79**:334-341

[23] Forster MC, Bruce AS, Aster AS. Should the tibia be reamed when nailing? Injury. 2005;**36**:439-444

[24] Study to Prospectively Evaluate Reamed Intramedullary Nails in Patients with Tibial Fractures Investigators, Bhandari M, Guyatt G, Tornetta P 3rd, et al. Randomized trial of reamed and unreamed intramedullary nailing of tibial shaft fractures. The Journal of Bone and Joint Surgery. 2008;**90**: 2567-2578. DOI: 10.2106/JBJS.G.01694

[25] Hull JB, Bell MJ. Modern trends for external fixation of fractures in children: A critical review. Journal of Pediatric Orthopaedics Part B. 1997;**6**:103-109

[26] Desai P, Audige L, Suk M. Combined orthopedic and vascular lower extremity injuries: Sequence of care and outcomes. American Journal of Orthopedics. 2012;**41**:182-186

[27] Stancic MF, Eskinja N, Bellinzona M, et al. The role of interfascular nerve grafting after gunshot wounds. A report of 44 cases. International Orthopaedics. 1996;**20**:87-91

[28] Mackinnon SE, Dellon AL. Clinical nerve reconstruction with a bioabsorbable polyglycolic acid tube. Plastic and Reconstructive Surgery. 1990;**85**:419-424

[29] MacKenzie EJ, Bosse MJ, Kellam JF, et al. Factors influencing the decision to amputate or reconstruct after high-energy lower extremity trauma. The Journal of Trauma. 2002;**52**:641-649

[30] Hertel R, Lambert SM, Muller S, et al. On the timing of soft-tissue reconstruction for open fractures of the lower leg. Archives of Orthopaedic and Trauma Surgery. 1999;**119**:7-12

[31] Hohmann E, Tetsworth K, Radziejowski MJ, Wiesniewski TF. Comparison of delayed and primary wound closure in the treatment of open tibial fractures. Archives of Orthopaedic and Trauma Surgery. 2007;**127**:131-136

[32] Jenkinson RJ, Kiss A, Johnson S, et al. Delayed wound closure increases

deep-infection rate associated with lower-grade open fractures: A propensity-matched cohort study. The Journal of Bone and Joint Surgery. 2014;**96**:380-386. DOI: 10.2106/JBJS.L.00545

[33] Stannard JP, Volgas DA, Stewart R, et al. Negative pressure wound therapy after severe open fractures: A prospective randomized study. Journal of Orthopaedic Trauma. 2009;**23**:552-557. DOI: 10.1097/BOT.0b013e3181a2e2b6

[34] Krug E, Berg L, Lee C, et al. Evidence-based recommendations for the use of negative pressure wound therapy in traumatic wounds and reconstructive surgery: Steps towards an international consensus. Injury. 2011;**42**(Suppl 1):S1-S12. DOI: 10.1016/S0020-1383(11)00041-6

[35] Iheozor-Ejiofor Z, Newton K, Dumville JC, et al. Negative pressure wound therapy for open traumatic wounds. Cochrane Database of Systematic Reviews. 3 Jul 2018;7:CD012522. DOI: 10.1002/14651858.CD012522.pub2

[36] Godina M. Early microsurgical reconstruction of complex trauma of the extremities. Plastic and Reconstructive Surgery. 1986;**78**:285-292

[37] D'Alleyrand JC, Manson TT, Dancy L, et al. Is time to flap coverage of open tibial fractures an independent predictor of flap-related complications? Journal of Orthopaedic Trauma. 2014;**28**:288-293. DOI: 10.1097/BOT.0000000000000001

[38] Gopal S, Majumder S, Batchelor AG, et al. Fix and flap: The radical orthopaedic and plastic treatment of severe open fractures of the tibia. Journal of Bone and Joint Surgery. 2000;**82**:959-966

[39] Pollak AN, McCarthy ML, Burgess AR. Short-term wound complications after application of flaps for coverage of traumatic soft-tissue defects about the tibia. The Lower Extremity Assessment Project (LEAP) Study Group. Journal of Bone and Joint Surgery. 2000;**82**:1681-1691

[40] Gopal S, Giannoudis PV, Murray A, et al. The functional outcome of severe, open tibial fractures managed with early fixation and flap coverage. Journal of Bone and Joint Surgery. 2004;**86**:861-867

[41] Webb LX, Bosse MJ, Castillo RC, MacKenzie EJ, LEAP Study Group. Analysis of surgeon-controlled variables in the treatment of limb-threatening type-III open tibial diaphyseal fractures. The Journal of Bone and Joint Surgery. 2007;**89**:923-928

[42] Nemoto M, Ishikawa S, Kounoike N, et al. Free flap transfer to preserve main arterial flow in early reconstruction of open fracture in the lower extremity. Plastic Surgery International. 2015;**2015**:213892. DOI: 10.1155/2015/213892

[43] Shackford SR, Davis JW, Hollingsworth-Fridlund P, et al. Venous thromboembolism in patients with major trauma. American Journal of Surgery. 1990;**159**:365-369

[44] Geerts WH, Code KI, Jay RM, et al. A prospective study of venous thromboembolism after major trauma. The New England Journal of Medicine. 1994;**331**:1601-1606

[45] Schultz DJ, Brasel KJ, Washington L, et al. Incidence of asymptomatic pulmonary embolism in moderately to severely injured trauma patients. The Journal of Trauma. 2004;**56**:727-731

[46] Rogers FB, Cipolle MD, Velmahos G, et al. Practice management guidelines for the prevention of venous thromboembolism in trauma patients: The EAST practice management

guidelines work group. The Journal of Trauma. 2002;**53**:142-164

[47] Francel TJ, Vander Kolk CA, Hoopes JE, et al. Microvascular soft-tissue transplantation for reconstruction of acute open tibial fractures: Timing of coverage and long-term functional results. Plastic and Reconstructive Surgery. 1992;**89**:478-489

[48] Hertel R, Strebel N, Ganz R. Amputation versus reconstruction in traumatic defects of the leg: Outcome and costs. Journal of Orthopaedic Trauma. 1996;**10**:223-229

[49] Chung KC, Saddawi-Konefka D, Haase SC, Kaul G. A cost-utility analysis of amputation versus salvage for Gustilo type IIIB and IIIC open tibial fractures. Plastic and Reconstructive Surgery. 2009;**124**:1965-1973. DOI: 10.1097/PRS.0b013e3181bcf156

[50] Fagelman MF, Epps HR, Rang M. Mangled extremity severity score in children. Journal of Pediatric Orthopedics. 2002;**22**:182-184

[51] Helfet DL, Howey T, Sanders R, Johansen K. Limb salvage versus amputation. Preliminary results of the Mangled Extremity Severity Score. Clinical Orthopaedics and Related Research. 1990;**256**:80-86

[52] Mommsen P, Zeckey C, Hildebrand F, et al. Traumatic extremity arterial injury in children: Epidemiology, diagnostics, treatment and prognostic value of mangled extremity severity score. Journal of Orthopaedic Surgery and Research. 2010;**5**:25. DOI: 10.1186/1749-799X-5-25

[53] Slauterbeck JR, Britton C, Moneim MS, Clevenger FW. Mangled extremity severity score: An accurate guide to treatment of the severely injured upper extremity. Journal of Orthopaedic Trauma. 1994;**8**:282-285

[54] Bonanni F, Rhodes M, Lucke JF. The futility of predictive scoring of mangled lower extremities. The Journal of Trauma. 1993;**34**:99-104

[55] Durham RM, Mistry BM, Mazuski JE, et al. Outcome and utility of scoring systems in the management of the mangled extremity. American Journal of Surgery. 1996;**172**:569-574

[56] Sheean AJ, Krueger CA, Napierala MA Skeletal Trauma and Research Consortium (STReC), et al.. Evaluation of the mangled extremity severity score in combat-related type III open tibia fracture. Journal of Orthopaedic Trauma 2014;**28**:523-526. DOI: 10.1097/BOT.0000000000000054

[57] Stewart DA, Coombs CJ, Graham HK. Application of lower extremity injury severity scores in children. Journal of Children's Orthopaedics. 2012;**6**:427-431. DOI: 10.1007/s11832-012-0439-6

[58] Brown KV, Ramasamy A, McLeod J, et al. Predicting the need for early amputation in ballistic mangled extremity injuries. The Journal of Trauma. 2009;**66**(4 Suppl):S93-S97. DOI: 10.1097/TA.0b013e31819cdcb0

[59] Doucet JJ, Galarneau MR, Potenza BM, et al. Combat versus civilian open tibia fractures: The effect of blast mechanism on limb salvage. The Journal of Trauma. 2011;**70**:1241-1247. DOI: 10.1097/TA.0b013e3182095b52

[60] Bosse MJ, MacKenzie EJ, Kellam JF, et al. A prospective evaluation of the clinical utility of the lower-extremity injury-severity scores. The Journal of Bone and Joint Surgery. 2001;**83**:3-14

Chapter 4

Scoring Systems in Major Extremity Traumas

Isil Akgun Demir and Semra Karsidag

Abstract

In the emergency room, every mangled extremity presents with its unique features. Each case requires a different approach and special care, while a surgeon has almost always the same facilities and armamentarium in her/his own setting. Thanks to the advancements in the bone fixation technologies and microsurgical field, the attempts to salvage mangled or even amputated limbs have increased. However, it is still controversial how the decision should be made for salvage or amputation. That is why several scoring systems have been proposed based on retrospective analysis of this group of patients in order to generate a systematic approach and to optimize the outcome. Although they help the surgeon to decide salvation over amputation, or vice versa, the same scores in different patient populations should be interpreted meticulously, and the treatment plan should be established accordingly. The ultimate success is being able to make the most accurate decision possible, and this can be only achieved with experience and extensive knowledge along with sufficient surgical skills.

Keywords: amputation, limb salvage, major trauma, mangled extremity, scoring system

1. Introduction

Approach to major limb traumas is still a challenging subject. The decision-making process is the most critical part directly affecting the outcome. Although several factors such as the general status of the patient, the condition of the limb, and the experience of the surgeon along with the availability of the facilities help greatly determining what to do next, the outcome is mostly unpredictable when it comes to salvaging of an injured or amputated limb.

The decision for salvation should be done only after it is confirmed that the patient has no accompanying life-threatening injuries. Once the patient is stable, then the injured or amputated limb should be examined thoroughly. If the injured part is grossly contaminated, is severely avulsed, or contains vascular injuries at multiple levels, the patient would not benefit from any salvage procedures; moreover, any attempt to salvage the limb might put the patient's life at risk.

The main concerns in this decision-making process focus on the extent of vascular, skeletal, and soft tissue damage, the presence of shock, and warm ischemia time. However, additional criteria such as age, contamination, and patient-related comorbidities cannot be disregarded. The details of the incident are also of great importance such as when it happened, the time interval between the incident and arrival to the hospital and mechanism of injury. Like in every patient presenting with major trauma, the initial evaluation should include the establishment of a patent airway and optimization of ventilation and blood circulation. After the patient is stabilized, a thorough physical examination should be performed. In patients presenting with mangled extremities, pulsation, skin color and temperature, and capillary return on the distal segment of the involved limb should be checked. If fracture or dislocation of the involved limb is suspected, X-ray or computed tomography images should be obtained. Peripheral nerve examination should be also performed prior to any intervention. Meanwhile, antibiotic therapy should be initiated as soon as possible, especially in case of open fracture, and tetanus prophylaxis must be administered immediately.

2. Scoring systems for upper and lower extremities

In order to be able to evaluate patients with major limb trauma in a more systematic way, several scoring systems have been proposed. The most widely used scoring systems are Mangled Extremity Syndrome Index (MESI); Mangled Extremity Severity Score (MESS); Predictive Salvage Index (PSI); Limb Salvage Index (LSI); Nerve injury, ischemia, soft tissue injury, skeletal injury, shock, age of patient score (NISSSA); and Ganga Hospital Open Injury Severity Scoring (GHOISS) (**Tables 1–6**).

Mangled Extremity Syndrome Index (**Table 1**) was described by Gregory et al. in 1985 [2]. The components of this index are injury severity score, bone, age, integument injury, nerve, lag time to operation, pre-existing disease, and shock. A cutoff score of 20 is considered for amputation.

Injury severity score	0–25	1
	25–50	2
	>50	3
Integument injury	Guillotine	1
	Crush/burn	2
	Avulsion/degloving	3
Nerve injury	Contusion	1
	Transection	2
	Avulsion	3
Vascular injury	Arterial transection	1
	Arterial thrombosis	2
	Arterial avulsion	3
	Vein	1
Bone injury	Simple	1
	Segmental	2
	Segmental comminuted	3
	Bone loss <6 cm	4
	Articular	5
	Articular with bone loss <6 cm	6
Age	<40 years	0
	40–50 years	1
	50–60 years	2
	>60 years	3
Lag time to operation	For each hour over 6 hours	1
Pre-existing disease		1
Shock		2

Table 1.
Mangled Extremity Severity Index (MESI).

Skeletal and soft tissue injury	Low-energy injury	1
	Medium-energy injury	2
	High-energy injury	3
	Very-high-energy injury or above injuries with gross contamination	4
Limb ischemia*	Normal perfusion despite reduced or non-palpable pulse	1
	Slow capillary refill	2
	No capillary refill	3
Shock status	Systolic blood pressure > 90 mm Hg	0
	Transient hypotension	1
	Persistent hypotension	2
Age	<30 years	0
	30–50 years	1
	>50 years	2

**The score is doubled if the warm ischemia time >6 hours.*

Table 2.
Mangled Extremity Severity Score (MESS).

Bone injury	Mild trauma	1
	Moderate trauma	2
	Severe trauma	3
Muscle injury	Mild trauma	1
	Moderate trauma	2
	Severe trauma	3
Arterial injury	Suprapopliteal	1
	Popliteal	2
	Infrapopliteal	3
Delay to the operating room	<6 hours	1
	6–12 hours	2
	>12 hours	3

Table 3.
Predictive salvage index (PSI).

MESS (**Table 2**) is probably the most commonly used scoring system worldwide for both upper and lower extremity traumas. It was developed by Johansen et al. in 1990 following a retrospective evaluation of patients with lower mangled extremities [3]. The criteria for MESS include age, the presence of shock, warm ischemia time, and skeletal and soft tissue injury. In case the warm ischemia time is longer than 6 hours, the score is doubled. A MESS value equal to or greater than 7 is suggested as highly predictive for amputation.

In 1987 PSI (**Table 3**) was proposed by Howe et al. for scoring lower extremities with orthopedic and vascular injury. In their study, they determined the cutoff value for amputation as 8 [4].

LSI (**Table 4**) was introduced by Russell et al. in 1991 [5]. Unlike the majority of scoring systems, age and the presence of shock are not included in LSI. On the other hand, there are seven evaluation criteria requiring extensive examination which can be only performed intraoperatively. A score of greater than 6 indicates amputation.

Artery	Contusion, intimal tear, partial laceration, or avulsion	0
	Occlusion of ≥2 leg vessels, non-palpable pedal pulses	1
	Complete occlusion of femoral or all three leg vessels	2
Nerve	Contusions, stretch injury, minimal clean laceration	0
	Partial transection or avulsion of sciatic nerve; complete/partial transection of femoral and peroneal/tibial nerve	1
	Complete transection/avulsion of sciatic nerve or both peroneal and tibial nerves	2
Bone	Closed fracture in ≤2 sites; open fracture without comminution; closed dislocation without fracture; fibula fracture; open joint without foreign body	0
	Closed fracture in at least three sites on same extremity; open fracture with comminution or moderate to large displacement; open joint with foreign body; bone loss <3 cm	1
	Bone loss >3 cm; Gustilo type IIIB,C fractures	2
Skin	Clean laceration or small avulsion injuries with primary repair or first-degree burn	0
	Delayed closure due to contamination; wounds requiring skin grafts or flaps; second- and third-degree burns	1
Muscle	Avulsion or laceration of a single compartment or single tendon	0
	Avulsion or laceration ≥2 compartments or tendons	1
	Crush injury	2
Deep vein	Contusion, partial laceration, or avulsion; complete laceration or avulsion with intact drainage; superficial vein injury	0
	Complete laceration, avulsion, or thrombosis without adequate venous drainage	1
Warm ischemia time	<6 hours	0
	6–9 hours	1
	9–12 hours	2
	12–15 hours	3
	>15 hours	4

Table 4.
Limb salvage index (LSI).

Nerve	Sensate	No major nerve injury	0
	Dorsal	Deep or superficial peroneal nerve injury	1
	Plantar partial	Tibial nerve injury	2
	Plantar complete	Sciatic nerve injury	3
Ischemia*	None	Good to fair pulses, no ischemia	0
	Mild	Reduced pulses, perfusion normal	1
	Moderate	No pulses, prolonged capillary refill, Doppler pulses present	2
	Severe	Pulseless, cool, ischemic, no Doppler pulses	3
Soft tissue	Low	Minimal to no contusion, no contamination	0
	Medium	Moderate injury, low-velocity gunshot wound, moderate contamination, minimal crush	1
	High	Moderate crush, deglove, high-velocity gunshot wound, moderate injury requiring flap, considerable contamination	2
	Severe	Massive crush, farm injury, severe deglove, severe contamination, requires flap	3
Skeletal	Low energy	Spiral fracture, oblique fracture, no or minimal displacement	0

	Medium energy	Transverse fracture, minimal comminution, small caliber gunshot wound	1
	High energy	Moderate displacement or comminution, high-velocity gunshot wound, butterfly fragments	2
	Severe energy	Segmental, severe comminution, bony loss	3
Shock	Normotensive	Blood pressure normal, always >90 mm Hg systolic	0
	Transient hypotension	Transient hypotension in field or emergency center	1
	Persistent hypotension	Persistent hypotension despite fluids	2
Age	Young	<30 years	0
	Middle	30–50 years	1
	Old	>50 years	2

Score doubles with ischemia >6 hours.

Table 5.
Nerve injury, ischemia, soft tissue, skeletal injury, shock, age of patient score (NISSSA) [6].

Covering structures: skin and fascia	*Wounds without skin loss*	Not over the fracture	1
		Exposing the fracture	2
	Wounds with skin loss	Not over the fracture	3
		Over the fracture	4
	Circumferential wound with skin loss		5
Skeletal structures: bone and joints	Transverse/oblique fracture/butterfly fragment <50%		1
	Large butterfly fragment >50% circumference		2
	Comminution/segmental fractures without bone loss		3
	Bone loss <4 cm		4
	Bone loss >4 cm		5
Functional tissues: MT and nerve units	Partial injury to MT unit		1
	Complete but repairable injury to MT units		2
	Irreparable injury to MT units/partial loss of a compartment/complete injury to posterior tibial nerve		3
	Loss of one compartment of MT units		4
	Loss of ≥2 compartments/subtotal amputation		5
Comorbid conditions	Drug-dependent diabetes mellitus/cardiorespiratory diseases leading to increased anesthetic risk		2
	Sewage or organic contamination/farmyard injuries		2
	Age > 65 years		2
	Injury-debridement interval > 12 hours		2
	Polytrauma involving the chest or abdomen with injury severity score > 25/ fat embolism		2
	Hypotension with systolic blood pressure < 90 mmHg at presentation		2
	Another major injury to the same limb/compartment syndrome		2

MT, musculotendinous unit.

Table 6.
The Ganga Hospital Injury Severity Score (GHOISS) [1].

NISSSA score (**Table 5**) was proposed by McNamara et al. in 1994 [6]. It is a modified version of MESS with the addition of nerve injury. The cutoff value of NISSSA for amputation is 11.

The latest scoring system GHOISS was introduced by Rajasekaran et al. in 2006 [1]. The purpose of the authors was to address the paucity of the current scoring systems in tibial injuries without a vascular deficit (Gustilo type IIIB). GHOISS has the maximum number of components when compared with the other scoring systems (**Table 6**). A score of 14 or below is favored for the salvation of the limb, whereas a score of 17 or above indicates amputation. The scores falling between 14 and 17 indicate "the gray zone."

3. Discussion

The scoring systems were developed to provide a systematic therapeutic approach to mangled extremities.

by grading the severity of an injury. Like every concept that tries to tidy up a complicated clinical scenario, these systems have advantages and disadvantages. Most of the scoring systems address lower extremity injuries, while there is no scoring system specifically designed for upper extremity [7]. A single scoring system cannot be established for both upper and lower extremities since they differ in terms of the amount of muscle bulk and the availability of vascular supply [8]. The warm ischemia time is the single factor that has a direct impact on the extent of tissue necrosis and ischemia-reperfusion injury. Thus, it is included in all scoring systems, as demonstrated in **Table 7**.

The most commonly used systems for upper extremity injuries are MESI and MESS [8, 9]. It has been suggested that MESI scoring is more reliable than MESS in terms of prediction of amputation in mangled upper extremity injuries [8]. However, in order to calculate the MESI score, a thorough examination must be completed, and all the accompanying injuries must be identified, which is time-consuming and precludes practicality. On the other hand, although MESS was criticized by several authors in terms of its accuracy and predictive value, it can be still used preoperatively in many clinical settings with ease [10, 11]. The advantage of MESS is that its calculation relies on inspection and basic examination and is reproducible.

	MESI	MESS	PSI	LSI	NISSSA	GHOISS
Age	✓	✓			✓	✓
Shock	✓	✓			✓	✓
Warm ischemia time	✓	✓	✓	✓	✓	✓
Bone injury	✓		✓	✓		✓
Muscle injury			✓	✓		✓
Skin injury	✓			✓		✓
Nerve injury	✓			✓	✓	
Deep vein injury				✓		
Skeletal/soft tissue		✓			✓	
Contamination					✓	✓
Time to treatment	✓			✓		
Co-morbidity	✓					✓

Table 7.
Comparison of the components of the scoring systems.

The severity of muscle and bone injuries in PSI is graded as mild, moderate, and severe. However, the limits differentiating the severity levels from each other were not described well. Hence it is quite confusing how to grade those injuries with PSI. It would also result in a subjective evaluation rather than a systematic and unbiased calculation [12].

The critic regarding NISSSA is that the severity of nerve injury is only based on the plantar surface sensation indicating the integrity of the tibial nerve, which is no more an absolute contraindication for limb salvage [1]. The sensitivity and specificity of NISSSA have also been found controversial [13].

GHOISS is the first system to describe "gray zone" clearly meaning the scores between 14 and 17. It has been suggested that the outcome of the injuries in the gray zone is dependent on noninjury factors such as the skill and experience of the surgical team, the availability of facilities, and the patient's request. GHOISS was reported to be useful in children as well [14]. In their series of 107 patients with type IIIB injury, Rajasekaran et al. have reported that the Ganga hospital score showed higher sensitivity and specificity for predicting amputation; however, as they have mentioned in their article, this must be validated with multicenter trials [1].

The absolute contraindications for limb salvage or in other words absolute indications for amputations are still open for discussion. Although there is no established consensus about this topic, the presence of certain factors may favor amputation over salvage. First of all, if the patient has an accompanying life-threatening injury, salvage procedure must not be attempted, and such situations render the scoring systems invalid. Another critical point is the warm ischemia time. Lange et al. have suggested that a crush injury with warm ischemia time longer than 6 hours is an absolute indication for amputation [7]. However, this cannot be applied to upper extremity injuries, since the upper extremity has less muscle bulk than the lower extremity and thus is less prone to develop ischemic injury [8]. Roessler et al. have put emphasis on the fluid balance and absence of a distal pulse on presentation that they are eventual indicators for amputation [12]; nevertheless, current advancements in both medical and surgical fields have overcome those concerns. Another historical indication for limb amputation was the nonfunctional posterior tibial nerve [7]. But, as the LEAP study group has demonstrated, the loss of plantar sensation is no more an indication for amputation [15]. Advanced age may also be included among the indications for primary amputation [16].

Albeit, these systems have been designed to enable the surgical team to make a decision, they are not 100% predictive of the ultimate outcome (salvage vs. amputation), and they are also not predictive of functional recovery among patients with successful extremity reconstruction [17–19]. The sensitivity and specificity rates are quite variable, and all the proposed scoring systems were found to be useful only to some extent [20]. Therefore, in addition to the scores calculated with these systems, patients must be evaluated along with injury pattern and pre-existing comorbidities, and the treatment should be planned also according to the patients' needs and demands. It is also imperative to take the experience and the skills of the microsurgeon into account. The optimal outcome would be achieved with a systematic multidisciplinary approach, availability of facilities, and always considering what is best for the patient. Raising high expectations both for the surgeon and the patient should be avoided. The technical and individual advancements in the microsurgical field cannot be overlooked; nevertheless, extreme attempts for limb salvage may be harmful to the patient. Moreover, it might become a huge burden for both sides in case it results in a nonfunctional extremity or requires secondary amputation. On the other hand, a patient can still prefer a nonfunctional but salvaged extremity, if there is no contraindication for performing salvage procedure. Therefore, patients' desire should also be considered as an additional subjective criterion during decision-making. In a nutshell, there is no single recommended scoring system either for upper or lower extremity injuries. They should be only utilized as guides during the planning of the treatment.

The decision for amputation should never be regarded as a failure. It would also be wise asking for consultation from more experienced colleagues before making the ultimate decision. It is the experience and the quality of clinical judgment that save the patient at the end of the day. The scoring systems are a collateral aid in this hard decision-making process. Their benefits are limited because they rely on retrospective data in small patient populations, and unfortunately it still seems to be unlikely to design a prospective model. What we can do better is to combine our experience, these proposed scoring systems for better interpretation of the scores, and narrowing the gray zone as much as possible. As Russel et al. put into words, "numbers cannot replace clinical judgment" [5].

4. Conclusion

Scoring systems are useful tools in the evaluation of patients with major extremity traumas. However, each patient requires an individual approach and would benefit from the surgeon's own experience.

Conflict of interest

The author declares no conflict of interest.

Author details

Isil Akgun Demir* and Semra Karsidag
University of Health Sciences, Sisli Hamidiye Etfal Training and Research Hospital, Plastic and Reconstructive Surgery, Istanbul, Turkey

*Address all correspondence to: isilakgundemir@gmail.com

References

[1] Rajasekaran S, Naresh Babu J, Sheenadhayalan J, Shetty AP, Sundararajan SR, Kumar M, et al. A score for predicting salvage and outcome in Gustilo type-IIIA and type-IIIB open tibial fractures. Journal of Bone and Joint Surgery. British Volume (London). 2006;**88**:1351-1360. DOI: 10.1302/0301-620X.88B10.17631

[2] Gregory RT, Gould RJ, Peclet M, Wagner JS, Gilbert DA, Wheeler JR, et al. The mangled extremity syndrome (M.E.S.): A severity grading system for multisystem injury of the extremity. The Journal of Trauma. 1985;**25**:1147-1150

[3] Johanesen K, Daines M, Howey T, Helfet D, Hansen ST Jr. Objective criteria accurately predict amputation following lower extremity trauma. The Journal of Trauma. 1990;**30**:568-572; discussion 572-573

[4] Howe HR Jr, Poole GV Jr, Hansen KJ, Clark T, Plonk GW, Koman LA, et al. Salvage of lower extremities following combined orthopedic and vascular trauma. A predictive salvage index. The American Surgeon. 1987;**53**:205-208

[5] Russell WL, Sailors DM, Whittle TB, Fisher DF Jr, Burns RP. Limb salvage versus traumatic amputation. A decision based on a seven-part predictive index. Annals of Surgery. 1991;**213**:473-480; discussion 480-481

[6] McNamara MG, Heckman JD, Corley FG. Severe open fractures of the lower extremity: A retrospective evaluation of the Mangled Extremity Severity Score (MESS). Journal of Orthopaedic Trauma. 1994;**8**:81-87

[7] Dirschl DR, Dahners LE. The mangled extremity: When should it be amputated? The Journal of the American Academy of Orthopaedic Surgeons. 1996;**4**:182-190

[8] Kumar RS, Singhi PK, Chidambaram M. Are we justified doing salvage or amputation procedure based on mangled extremity severity score in mangled upper extremity injury. Journal of Orthopaedic Case Reports. 2017;**7**: 3-8. DOI: 10.13107/jocr.2250-0685.662

[9] Durham RM, Mistry BM, Mazuski JE, Shapiro M, Jacobs D. Outcome and utility of scoring systems in the management of the mangled extremity. American Journal of Surgery. 1996;**172**:569-573; discussion 573-574. DOI: 10.1016/S0002-9610(96)00245-0

[10] Prasarn ML, Helfet DL, Kloen P. Management of the mangled extremity. Strategies in Trauma and Limb Reconstruction. 2012;**7**:57-66. DOI: 10.1007/s11751-012-0137-4

[11] Loja MN, Sammann A, DuBose J, Li CS, Liu Y, Savage S, et al. The mangled extremity score and amputation: Time for a revision. Journal of Trauma and Acute Care Surgery. 2017;**82**:518-523. DOI: 10.1097/TA.0000000000001339

[12] Roessler MS, Wisner DH, Holcroft JW. The mangled extremity. When to amputate? Archives of Surgery. 1991;**126**:1243-1248; discussion 1248-1249

[13] Karna MB. Retrospective study on predictive scoring system for amputation in open fracture of tibia type III. International Journal of Research in Medical Sciences. 2016;**4**:3521-3524. DOI: 10.18203/2320-6012.ijrms20162323

[14] Venkatadass K, Grandhi TSP, Rajasekaran S. Use of Ganga Hospital Open Injury Severity scoring for determination of salvage versus amputation in open type IIIB injuries of lower limbs in children—An analysis of 52 type IIIB open fractures. Injury. 2017;**48**:2509-2514. DOI: 10.1016/j.injury.2017.09.010

[15] Bosse MJ, McCarthy ML, Jones AL, Webb LX, Sims SH, Sanders RW, et al. The insensate foot following severe lower extremity trauma: An indication for amputation? The Journal of Bone and Joint Surgery. American Volume. 2005;**87**:2601-2608. DOI: 10.2106/JBJS.C.00671

[16] Ninkovic M, Voigt S, Dornseifer U, Lorenz S, Ninkovic M. Microsurgical advances in extremity salvage. Clinics in Plastic Surgery. 2012;**39**:491-505. DOI: 10.1016/j.cps.2012.08.003

[17] Schirò GR, Sessa S, Piccioli A, Maccauro G. Primary amputation vs limb salvage in mangled extremity: A systematic review of the current scoring system. BMC Musculoskeletal Disorders. 2015;**16**:372. DOI: 10.1186/s12891-015-0832-7

[18] Ly TV, Travison TG, Castillo RC, Bosse MJ, MacKenzie EJ, LEAP Study Group. Ability of lower-extremity injury severity scores to predict functional outcome after limb salvage. The Journal of Bone and Joint Surgery. American Volume. 2008;**90**:1738-1743. DOI: 10.2106/JBJS.G.00136

[19] Bonanni F, Rhodes M, Lucke JF. The futility of predictive scoring of mangled lower extremities. The Journal of Trauma. 1993;**34**:99-104

[20] Bosse MJ, MacKenzie EJ, Kellam JF, Burgess AR, Webb LX, Swiontkowski MF, et al. A prospective evaluation of the clinical utility of the lower-extremity injury-severity scores. The Journal of Bone and Joint Surgery. American Volume. 2001;**83**:3-14

Chapter 5

Stump Overgrowth after Limb Amputation in Children

Rami Jahmani and Dror Paley

Abstract

Stump overgrowth is the most common complication after limb amputation in children. Its morbidity is relatively high, that required frequent revisions of the stump and prosthesis. The incidence of stump overgrowth varies in the literature; depending on different factors. The exact pathogenesis is unclear, many hypotheses have been suggested. The treatment is a challenge; simple excision of the bone is associated with recurrence and further shorting of the stump. Many options of treatment have been used. This paper is an up-to date literature review that includes the definition, incidence, pathogenesis, clinical presentation, radiographic diagnosis, and treatment options of stump overgrowth in children.

Keywords: limb amputation, stump overgrowth, complication of amputation, stump capping procedures, heterotopic ossification

1. Introduction

Overgrowth is the most common complication after stump amputation in children, and it leads to significant morbidity and multiple revisions of both the stump and prosthesis [1–3]. Overgrowth is characterized by the formation of bone spikes at the end of the amputated stump. At some point, the bone end becomes covered with a bursa, and skin adheres to the underlying bone. Finally, the skin perforates, and bone and soft tissue infections develop, **Figure 1**.

2. Incidence

Stump overgrowth is the most common complication following limb amputation in children, and the incidence varies from 4 to 50% [2–8]. Age, location, reason for amputation, and level of amputation are known factors that affect the prevalence of stump overgrowth. Among them age and location are the most influencing factors. Osseous overgrowth is not observed in children older than 12 years or in cases of disarticulation amputations. Younger patients have a higher incidence of stump overgrowth [1, 7, 9]. The most frequent locations are the humerus, followed by the fibula and the tibia, whereas stump overgrowth is rare in the radius and ulna [7, 10]. Traumatic amputations carry a higher risk of overgrowth than elective surgical amputations, as stump overgrowth is very rare in congenital agenesis but common in amniotic band syndrome [1–3, 5, 11, 12].

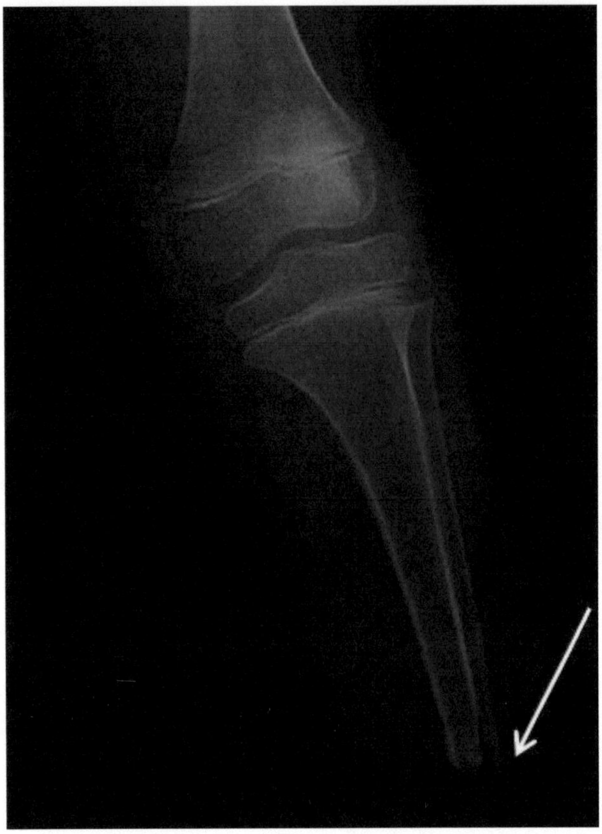

Figure 1.
X-ray of distal tibia and fibula overgrowth, arrow is indicating the sharp end of overgrown spike.

Aitke postulated that bone overgrowth in congenital cases is due to intrauterine amputation (amniotic band syndrome) rather than true agenesis, considering that bone overgrowth does not occur in congenital agenesis; however, this assumption has not been proven [7]. An increased prevalence of overgrowth has been reported in patients who had previously undergone surgery for overgrowth [3, 11, 12]. Last, metaphyseal level amputations carry a higher risk of overgrowth than diaphyseal level amputations [1, 5].

3. Pathogenesis

Many hypotheses have been proposed to explain the phenomenon of bone overgrowth. Because overgrowth occurs in children, it has been suggested that overgrowth occurs as a result of disproportional growth between the remaining proximal physis and the contracted distal soft tissue and skin [13–15]. Pellicore et al. observed bone growth stimulation following amputation and concluded that stump overgrowth occurs because soft tissues cannot keep up with the rapid growth of the bone [16]; however, attempts to treat overgrowth by proximal epiphysiodesis and leaving long redundant soft tissue have failed [12, 17–19]. The incidence of the overgrowth phenomenon in cases of surgical and post-trauma amputations was higher [1–3, 5] compared with that of disarticulation amputation and congenital agenesis, [7, 20] which suggests that stump overgrowth might be a result of bone and soft tissue trauma rather than continuous growth of the proximal physis. This would mean that overgrowth is a local

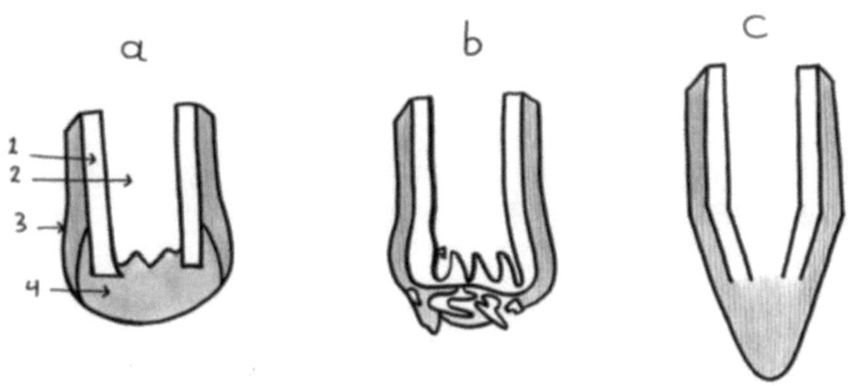

Figure 2.
Pathogenesis of stump overgrowth: (a) initial stage, hematoma formation and periosteal elevation. (b) Organization of collagen fibers of scar and periosteum as continues mass. (c) Pulling the collagen fibers more distal by wound contracture and spike formation. 1 – Cotrex, 2 – Medullary canal, 3 – Periosteum, 4 – Hematoma.

process of bone formation and wound healing that occur in the distal stump. Studying the histology of stump overgrowth in rabbits, Hellstadius concluded that the medullary canal is the source of overgrowth [21]. Aitken implanted a radiographic marker in the bony stump and confirmed that overgrowth occurs distal to the marker, proving that overgrowth does not represent an epiphyseal contribution but rather a local phenomenon of bone healing [7, 8]. This explains why overgrowth does not occur in cases of disarticulation where there is intact articular cartilage rather than transected bone. If stump overgrowth is a local phenomenon, it is unclear why it is not observed following adult amputation. Speer, by conducting an experimental histological study on the immature skeleton of rabbits, described the pathogenesis of stump overgrowth and explained why it does not occur in the mature skeleton [22]. His study indicates that an amputation stump responds via wound healing and intramembranous bone formation. In the immature skeleton, the elastic characteristic of the periosteum allows it to pull away from the end of the amputee stump and leads to local bone formation, **Figure 2**.

4. Diagnosis and clinical picture

Patients with stump overgrowth present with pain, intolerance to the prosthesis, soft tissue irritation, pressure ulcers, skin perforation, and infection. The sharp edge of the bony spike can be palpated subcutaneously. The diagnosis is confirmed radiographically, with characteristic distal tapering of the bone to a narrow tip, with the absence of a medullary canal (the so-called licked candy sign), **Figure 1**. Orthopaedists should differentiate between stump overgrowth and bone spurs, which develop as a response to periosteal stimulation at the periphery of transected bone edges. Such bone spurs rarely necessitate stump revision. The cause of pain might also be an adventitious bursa, which is common in soft tissues overlying an area of the stump.

5. Treatment

5.1 Conservative treatment

The initial management of stump overgrowth includes prosthetic modifications and lifestyle adjustments. Before wearing the prosthesis, soft tissues should be pulled distally to prevent "mushrooming" of the soft tissue proximally into the socket. In many cases, the cause of pain is attributed to bone spurs and adventitious bursae, which can be treated with aspiration, steroid injections, and stump wrapping.

The skin traction method, first described by Marquardt in the late 1960s, has been reported to be successful in selected cases [10, 23]. This method has become the standard in very young children with very short stumps, in whom further shortening may preclude the use of prosthetics. The method involves a lengthy treatment and requires a cooperative parent. Older children can be taught to apply traction by themselves. The early period at the beginning of the treatment, before the skin becomes adherent to the underlying bursa, is important. The method is less successful for amputations below the knee due to the presence of the interosseous membrane and related tissue that hold the soft tissue firmly to the bone. Traction should be applied 23 hours a day, with 1 hour off for cleaning, and should be continued until skeletal maturity. A skin adhesive, such as Hollister medical skin adhesive, is applied to the distal stump. Cotton or nylon stockinettes are placed on the limb over the adhesive and pressed onto the skin firmly. After the adhesive dry, the loose end of the fabric is split into medial and lateral "tails." The tails are cut to the skin margin where the stockinette is adherent to the skin and are used to counter-pull through a D-ring attached to the outside of the socket after being looped around a rod built into the prosthesis. Night traction is achieved by attaching the tail of the stockinette to rob with appropriate weight over a pulley on the side of the bed.[1]

5.2 Surgical treatment

The surgical treatment of stump overgrowth has always been a challenge. Simple excision of the overgrown bone is associated with high recurrence; Davids et al. [11] reported a rate of revision as high as 87% after simple bone excision, multiple revisions (more than one revision) have been reported in 18% of cases, and one case with six revisions has been reported [5, 12]. Repeated surgical excision, while it is temporarily effective, leads to progressive shortening of the stump. A lack of understanding of the pathogenesis has led to a wide variety of treatment recommendations. Disproportional growth between bone and soft tissue has been considered a reason for overgrowth in the immature skeleton. Attempts to treat the condition by proximal epiphysiodesis and leaving a redundant soft tissue envelope have failed to stop overgrowth [12, 17–19]. The recent hypothesis, which considers overgrowth a local appositional overgrowth as a result of the healing process [6–8, 21], has directed surgical treatment for reducing the intensity of the bone healing process. Attempts to stop local bone formation by sclerosing the end of the stump by periosteal excision and cauterization have failed to treat the condition, and histological studies of the excised-periosteum distal stump have shown viable bony tissue [3]. To interrupt the interaction between the endosteum and surrounding outside soft and bony tissues, capping of the medullary canal has been suggested. The first capping procedure was performed by Swanson in 1969 with the use of silicon rubber [24, 25]. Marquardt, in 1974, has been credited as being the first to propose the application of a biological cap to prevent bone overgrowth in children. He described his procedure of using an epiphysis taken from the amputated limb as a cap to prevent overgrowth of a distal tibia amputation [26]. The goal was to convert a diaphyseal amputation into a stump resembling a disarticulation type, **Figure 3**. Many animal and human studies have been conducted to study the result of capping procedures using different materials, including 1 – biological caps: cancellous, cortical, and cartilaginous caps from the amputated distal stump and iliac crest; and

[1] The technique is furthered described in [23].

2 – synthetic caps: rubber, polyethylene, titanium, and Teflon caps [1, 3, 4, 11, 24, 26–32] (**Table 1**). Animal studies on rabbits, with transplantation of the metatarsal epiphyses and fixation to the end of the amputated bone, have shown epiphyseal capping to be a very successful procedure to prevent overgrowth [31]. Many further publications have shown capping of the stump with an osteochondral cap to be the most effective treatment, with a revision rate of 0–10% [4, 29, 32, 33]. A controlled study compared osteochondral capping of the stump with simple resection and found a revision rate of 10% and, subsequently, of 86% [11, 28]. The distal epiphysis of the amputated stump, distal tibia, distal ulna, head of the metatarsal bone, and calcaneus serve as donors for the osteochondral cap for primary amputation (amputation where a distal stump is available). Finding a donor for the osteochondral cap is a challenge in secondary amputation (revision cases and cases where the distal part is absent), and the proximal fibula of the ipsilateral knee can be used in these situations [4, 29, 31, 33]. To avoid donor site morbidity (knee instability), Paley D used the apophysis of the iliac crest as a cap in a case series of patients [34]. Bernd et al. [27] studied the relationship between the revision rate in cartilaginous stump plasty and different factors and found no relationship with sex, reason for amputation, origin of the graft or method of fixation (screw vs. wires). However, revision was related to age and site; there were no revisions in patients below the age of 10 years old, and there were more revisions in the humerus; the high revision rate in the humerus was attributed to a loose interference fit between the humeral shaft and cartilaginous cap [32].

To avoid donor site morbidity and to substitute biological caps when unavailable, synthetic cap usage has been attractive for orthopedist. Silicon rubber, polyethylene and titanium caps have shown poor results [3, 11, 24]. Although capping

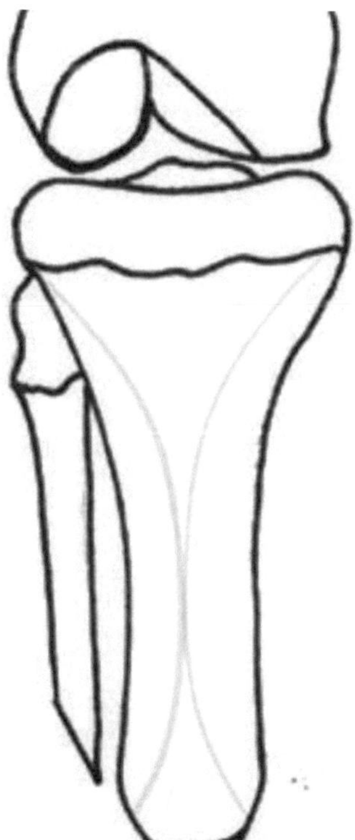

Figure 3.
Tibia stump plugged by cartilaginous cap.

N	Year	Author	Revision rate	Type of cap	Note
1	1978	Wang et al.	Zero	Epiphyseal cap from amputated limb of rabbits	Animal study
2	1991	Bernd et al.	12%	Bone graft	
3	1992	Benevenia et al.	10%	Epiphyseal cap form amputated segment	
4	1992	Hugh et al.	Zero	Ipsilateral fibula	
5	1995	Davids et al.	70%	Polyethellene	Failure mainly due to infection, prosthesis loosening, difficult soft tissue coverage
6	1995	Davids et al.	27%	Bone graft	
7	2004	Davids et al.	29%	Teflon	
8	2015	Fedorak et al.	10%	Ipsilateral fibula transplanted to tibias	
9	2017	Fedorak et al.	30%	Ipsilateral fibula transplanted to humerii	High failure rate in humerii treated by osteochondral transplantation
10	2017	Fedorak et al.	69%	Bone graft	
11	2019	Paley and Jahmani	50%	Apophysis of the ileac crest	A case series

Table 1.
Result of caping procedure by different authors using different capping materials.

with synthetic material is successful for reducing the intensity of bony growth, the revision rate is high because of failure of fixation, infection, implant fracture, and difficulty covering with soft tissue. The synthetic cap must be biologically inert and durable. Teflon caps show better results than other synthetic materials, with a 29% revision rate. This result is comparable to capping of the stump with bone grafts; the cause of failure is mainly due to infection and painful bursa rather than overgrowth [3].

Conclusion of treatment: conservative treatment (prosthesis and lifestyle modification) is the initial treatment, and the skin traction method can be used in selected cases, especially in very young patients and cases of short stumps. When performing amputations, prophylactic transplantation of an osteochondral graft to plug the stump is recommended when a graft is available. In revision cases and cases in which the osteochondral graft is unavailable, the head of the fibula and Teflon caps can be used to plug the stump.

Acknowledgements

The authors are thankful to Maha Almaani for drawing the figures.

Author details

Rami Jahmani[1*] and Dror Paley[2]

1 Department of Special Surgery/Orthopaedic Division, Faculty of Medicine, Jordan University of Science and Technology, Irbid, Jordan

2 Paley Orthopedic and Spine Institute, St. Mary's Hospital, West Palm Beach, Florida, USA

*Address all correspondence to: dr.Jahmany@yahoo.com

References

[1] Michels F, De Smet L. Osseous overgrowth in congenital amputations of the upper limb: Report of 3 cases treated with autologous stump plasty. Acta Orthopaedica Belgica. 2001;**67**(5):452-455

[2] Vocke AK, Schmid A. Osseous overgrowth after post-traumatic amputation of the lower extremity in childhood. Archives of Orthopaedic and Trauma Surgery. 2000;**120**(7-8):452-454

[3] Tenholder M, Davids JR, Gruber HE, Blackhurst DW. Surgical management of juvenile amputation overgrowth with a synthetic cap. Journal of Pediatric Orthopedics. 2004;**24**(2):218-226

[4] Fedorak GT, Watts HG, Cuomo AV, Ballesteros JP, Grant HJ, Bowen RE, et al. Osteocartilaginous transfer of the proximal part of the fibula for osseous overgrowth in children with congenital or acquired tibial amputation: Surgical technique and results. Journal of Bone and Joint Surgery. 2015;**1, 97**(7):574-581

[5] O'Neal M, Bahner R, Geney T, Ogden J. Osseous overgrowth after amputation in adolescents and children. Journal of Pediatric Orthopedics. 1996;**16-A**:78-84

[6] Abraham E, Pellicore RJ, Hamilton RC, Hallman BW, Ghosh L. Stump overgrowth in juvenile amputees. Journal of Pediatric Orthopedics. 1986;**6**:66-71

[7] Aitken G. Surgical amputation in children. Journal of Bone and Joint Surgery. 1963;**45**:1735-1741

[8] Aitken G. Overgrowth of the amputation stump. Inter Clinic Information Bulletin. 1962;**1**:1

[9] Abraham E. Operative treatment of bone overgrowth in children who have an acquired or congenital amputation (letter). Journal of Bone and Joint Surgery. 1996;**78**:1287-1288

[10] Atkins D, Meier R. Comprehensive Management of the Upper-Limb Amputee. 3rd ed. New York: Springer-verlag; 1989

[11] Davids JR, Meyer LC, Blackhurst DW. Operative treatment of bone overgrowth in children who have an acquired or congenital amputation. Journal of Bone and Joint Surgery. 1995;**77**:1490-1497

[12] Pfeil J, Marquardt E, Holtz T, Niethard FU, Schneider E, Carstens C. The stump capping procedure to prevent or treat terminal osseous overgrowth. Prosthetics and Orthotics International. 1991;**15**(2):96-99

[13] Beekman F. Amputations during childhood. The Surgical Clinics of North America. 1938;**18**:425

[14] Frantz A, Aitken G. Management of the juvenile amputee. Clinical Orthopaedics. 1959;**14**:30

[15] Kurtz A, Hand R. Bone growth following amputation in childhood. American Journal of Surgery. 1939;**43**:773

[16] Pellicore RJ, Sciora J, Lambert CN, Hamilton RC. Incidence of bone overgrowth in the juvenile amputee population. Inter Clinic Information Bulletin. 1974;**13**:1-10

[17] Saal F. Epiphysiodesis combined with amputation. Journal of Bone and Joint Surgery. 1939;**21**:442

[18] Aitken GT. The child with an acquired amputation. Inter Clinic Information Bulletin. 1968;**7**:1-15

[19] Drvaric DM, Kruger LM. Modified Ertl osteomyoplasty for terminal

overgrowth in childhood limb deficiencies. Journal of Pediatric Orthopedics. 2001;**21**:392-394

[20] Firth GB, Masquijo JJ, Kontio K. Transtibial Ertl amputation for children and adolescents: A case series and literature review. Journal of Children's Orthopaedics. 2011;**5**(5):357-362. DOI: 10.1007/s11832-011-0364-0

[21] Hellstadius A. An investigation, by experiments on animals, of the role played by the epiphysial cartilage in longitudinal growth. Acta Chirurgica Scandinavica. 1947;**95**:156

[22] Speer DP. The pathogenesis of amputation stump overgrowth. Clinical Orthopaedics and Related Research. 1981;(159):294-307

[23] Friedmann LW, Friedmann L. The conservative treatment of the bony overgrowth problem in the juvenile amputee. Inter Clinic Information Bulletin. 1985;**20**(2):17-23

[24] Swanson AB. Bone overgrowth in the juvenile amputee and its control by the use of silicone rubber implants. Inter Clinic Information Bulletin. 1969;**8**:9-18

[25] Swanson AB. Silicone-rubber implants to control the overgrowth phenomenon in the juvenile amputee. Inter Clinic Information Bulletin. 1972;**11**:5-8

[26] Marquardt E. Plastische Operationen bei drohender Knochendurchspießung am kindlichen Oberarmstumpf. Zeitschrift für Orthopädie. 1976;**114**:711-714

[27] Bernd L, Blasius K, Lukoschek M, Lücke R. The autologous stump plasty. Treatment for bony overgrowth in juvenile amputees. Journal of Bone and Joint Surgery. 1991;**73**:203-206

[28] Davids JR. Terminal bony overgrowth of the residual limb: Current management strategies. In: Herring JA, Birch JG, editors. The Child with a Limb Deficiency. Rosemont, IL: The American Academy of Orthopaedic Surgeons; 1998. pp. 269-280

[29] Benevenia J, Makley JT, Leeson MC, Benevenia K. Primary epiphyseal transplantsand bone overgrowth in childhood amputations. Journal of Pediatric Orthopedics. 1992;**12**:746-750

[30] Meyer LC, Sauer BW. The use of porous high-density polyethylene caps in the prevention of appositional bone growth in the juvenile amputee: A preliminary report. Inter Clinic Information Bulletin. 1975;**14**:1

[31] Wang G-J, Baugher WH, Stamp WG. Epiphyseal transplant in amputations. Effects on overgrowth in a rabbit Model. Clinical Orthopaedics and Related Research. 1978;(130):285-288

[32] Fedorak GT, Cuomo AV, Watts HG, Scaduto AA. Management of terminal osseous overgrowth of the humerus with simple resection and osteo-cartilaginous grafts. Journal of Pediatric Orthopedics. 2017;**37**(3):e216-ee22

[33] Hugh GW, Yoshio S. Marquardt stump capping for overgrowth. Journal of the Association of Children's Prosthetic & Orthotic Clinics. 1992;**27**:6

[34] Jahmani R, Robbins C, Paley D. Iliac crest apophysis transfer to treat stump overgrowth after limb amputation in children: Case series and literature review. International Orthopaedics. 2019. DOI: 10.1007/s00264-019-04289-y. [Epub ahead of print]